To Billie

with all good wishes
for your health &

happiness.

Mary

Flying in the Face of Fear

Mary Lunnen

Mary Lunnen

The Hypatia Trust
Newmill
1998

Published for the Hypatia Trust by the Patten Press 1998

This book is dedicated to Mikki

Table of Contents

Explanations of technical terms can be found in the glossary on page 114.

Foreword

It is devastating to be told you have cancer -- or that someone you love has. Being given such a diagnosis affects patients and their families in a myriad of ways. The only sure thing is that nothing is ever the same again and many people feel that their life has been turned upside down as they face their own mortality. Cervical cancer can be particularly traumatic for women as surgery, generally the primary treatment for the disease, cuts to the very heart of what being a woman means.

When given a diagnosis of a potentially life-threatening disease, a patient is compelled to make difficult decisions about treatment. Generally, patients know little about the fine detail of how their body works and what the real impact of any treatment will be. Suddenly they are placed in the position of having to find out about the things that will influence their decision and about the key aspects of the treatments.

No one knows just how an individual will respond to treatment, nor what the future holds. Talking through fears and uncertainties with someone who understands how you feel, but is outside the circle of friends and family, provides an important support at a stressful time. Organisations such as CancerBACUP offer the opportunity to do just that, and Mary Lunnen herself found how helpful it is to be able to pick up the phone and speak directly to a supportive and compassionate nurse, able to answer any question however trivial it might seem.

One of the ways that many women help themselves come to terms with cancer is to talk to other women who have had the same illness -- and come through it. It is immensely reassuring to know that you are not the only person to have suffered from cervical cancer and to find that many women not only survive it but continue to lead full and satisfying lives, having recovered from the disease. This book gives women's personal accounts of how they have faced the diagnosis and treatment and it will allow patients and their families to draw strength from the individual histories.

Jean Mossman
Chief Executive, CancerBACUP
April 1998

Thanks & acknowledgements

My sincere thanks to all contributors to this book, for their stories, and their encouragement throughout the time spent on its 'birth' and to Eric for the inspiring and so appropriate title. Special thanks to the sponsors, Mr K.E. Millward of Leo Pharmaceuticals, Delia and Adrian Read, Brain Mulrooney, Carol McKeough, Rita Johnson and friends who wish to remain anonymous.

To Melissa Hardie and all at the Patten Press, for support, good advice, and special skills.

To Jean Mossman, Anne-Marie Jones, all at CancerBACUP and all friends who have had faith in this book from the beginning of the idea.

To my husband and family, in the UK and New Zealand, for love, patience and understanding.

Introduction

On 12 May 1994 I sat in shock in my GP's surgery as she told me that I had cervical cancer and required a radical hysterectomy and possibly radiotherapy. One of my first questions was "Can I speak to someone else who has been through this?"

My doctor's reply was that she could not give me any names due to patient confidentiality. I have since discovered that some GPs and hospitals keep a register of volunteers who are prepared to help other women in this way. This book is an attempt to help those who find themselves in my situation - and their families, friends and carers - by telling the stories of women who have been through the terrible experience of diagnosis and treatment for cervical cancer.

When I looked for help in that fearful week following diagnosis, I found various helplines and information services (particularly BACUP -- now CancerBACUP) extremely helpful with support, and in explaining medical terms, but none of these dealt specifically with cervical cancer.

I am grateful to the people (many of them readers of CancerBACUP News) who have volunteered to tell their stories for this book. Everyone's experience is different and no one now going through treatment for this disease will have exactly the same symptoms, treatment, feelings, fears, as anyone else, but just hearing others 'talk' who have gone through it is a great comfort. Some family members and friends have also contributed, I am sure these accounts will be valuable to those trying to come to terms with the fact that their loved ones have been diagnosed with cancer.

The stories told here contain all the individualities of women's lives and backgrounds. Reactions to the diagnosis are different and so are the outcomes -- and so are coping strategies. Some people turn to complementary medicine, religion, meditation; some try to go back to exactly how they were before cancer affected them; some change their lives completely.

Medically, there is no answer for the question 'why me?', though many people believe that cancers are more likely to strike those who are under stress, either mental or physical, or both. Whatever the truth of this, many of the participants in this book have used their illness as a chance to reflect on things they wish to change in their lives, and in some cases have made radical alterations to how they live.

I have been moved by the willingness of these women to talk and share their experiences, and also by the courage, humour and optimism with which they have faced (and are still facing) such a frightening experience. The stories will have different meanings for every reader, there are sad and difficult moments, but also inspiring and encouraging ones. Not everyone may wish to take up wing-walking like Delia, but her photograph on the cover of this book dramatically illustrates that we can all achieve our ambitions.

All of us who have had to live with cancer know that it changes your life for ever. If this book can help others in at least a small way to see that there is a way through the fog of darkness and despair to the light - whether that be full recovery, coping with a continuing illness, or finding a way to make your peace with the world before you leave it - we will have been able to pass on the gifts that have been given us by our survival.

The main part of this book is made up of the stories of the contributors, mostly in their own words -- who better to tell of their experiences than themselves? Then I have drawn together and discussed some of the points that emerge, with a glossary of terms. The appendices contain a summary of advice, contact addresses and other reading that may be useful.

This book is dedicated to all who have participated, and particularly to the memory of Mikki who offered to contribute her story even whilst in the middle of treatment, but who tragically died before the book was completed. Although I have not included her story in full, the Afterword contains extracts with some important points she wanted to make, together with contributions from her husband and a close friend.

Note: please refer to your doctor with any queries about your own treatment, or before embarking on complementary therapies. These personal accounts are written from memory by ordinary people without (on the most part) any specialist knowledge.

Bernadette's story

I am 69 now, with three adult sons and two grand-daughters. My husband is a retired design engineer. I spend a lot of time involved with music - playing piano for ballet classes, and electric organ at a spiritualist church. My spiritual conviction was the direct result of receiving wonderful spiritual healing from Doug and Vera Bateman (the original healers for our group). I was so excited to hear messages and information from the spirit world coming through for people who instantly knew who was making contact - what a wonderful revelation that is!

I had a hysterectomy in 1987, two years after my diagnosis. This was following a routine smear test, but I was not given the result for three and a half months! I began by trying to use natural medicine because I was totally petrified of hospitals and surgeons, even though at the beginning it need only have been a simple biopsy and laser treatment.

When I discovered the Northumberland Cancer Support Group, I was so relieved to find people to talk to and be with. The group was set up as a support for the Bristol Cancer Help Centre. Joan Ridley, our founder, had spent a week there, and was keen to take some of the love and support provided there and offer it to people in the north of England. As I was really quite blown apart by the constant pull from my doctor, and local hospital, I needed very much to 'get my head sorted out'. So Joan, the very next day, got in touch with Bristol, and I was offered £300 from their bursary fund towards the cost of our stay.

It was an unforgettable experience and every day I was able to work through my many and various hang-ups about hospitals, anaesthetics, etc. in the wonderful relaxation and visualisation sessions we experienced. At the end of the week my doctor at the Bristol Centre told me that he had talked with my GP (having sought my permission beforehand), and that the picture was quite bleak. I was by then in the third stage of the cancerous condition, and at any time it could develop into something much more serious.

And so, by then having had the wonderful support of loving healers, and friends at home, with the so-effective therapies at Bristol, I was a very different person, and was able to return home, phone my GP, and say "OK -- go ahead."

I was told I needed a hysterectomy -- uterus and ovaries, but I feel that I had been given those two years so that I could become so much stronger spiritually and mentally. The operation went well and I was so calm about it all. The care in hospital was superb -- I just have good, and funny memories, even eleven years later!

The spiritual side of life interests me a great deal. I am sure that there is life after death because, firstly, I have heard and read so much evidence of this. Secondly, the knowledge that we go back to the spirit world when we leave our earthly shells makes so much sense to me. Also, that we have lived many lives before, and can choose to return again to 'learn more lessons', to enable us to progress, makes even more sense. (But I never ask people to accept these views unless they feel they can do so!). I also understand that we are all on different levels of our eternal existence, which explains why we all vary so much in our outlook on life.

The Northumberland Cancer Support Group is just fantastic, and more and more people are joining and attending regularly. We offer reflexology, aromatherapy, Reiki healing, and counselling every week, and visit members at home or in hospital. We also support carers as well as patients. We meet every Tuesday evening and have the use of a good building, with separate rooms for use by the various therapists.

We enjoy talks and demonstrations given by a variety of interesting people -- yoga, tai chi, nutrition, health kinesiology, Alexander technique. Also we hold weekend workshops e.g. Healing Touch, Death and Dying, Tai Chi. A good number of us attend the annual Cancer Conference in Manchester each year and have a wonderful and enlightening four days, the effects of which stay with us for ever. Last autumn 35 of us had a brilliant weekend at Kirkby Fleetham in Yorkshire, which was of great benefit to us all. I am not a 'committee person', but I go along as an enthusiastic supporter and help out by collecting and returning keys the next morning. The Group is a very important part of my life!

Contact: Linda Brinkhurst (Secretary/Chairman), 47 Apperley Road, Stocksfield, Northumberland,Tel: 01661 842919

"I'm only in this for life" - Beverley's story

When I was informed that I had adenocarcinoma of the cervix in June 1996, I had not had any relevant symptoms, though my periods were becoming lighter and I did start to bleed very slightly after intercourse. I thought I had more chance of winning the lottery than getting cancer of the cervix.

At that time I had been trying for another child, as my daughter was nearly three years old. As I had not become pregnant I went to see my GP, he did not seem concerned and told me not to worry, as it can take up to 12 months. I decided to see another GP within the surgery, who, after doing a smear test, made an appointment for me to see a gynaecologist.

As I was a private patient I was seen after about two weeks for a colposcopy. I received a letter after this appointment for a follow-up consultation. As it was the last appointment of the week, I was not unduly concerned, as if it had been serious I felt sure I would have been given an earlier appointment in that week. I was given no advance warning that it was bad news, so I attended by myself. I feel that I should have received an earlier appointment, and that I should have been told that it was preferable that I did not attend alone. It wasn't handled very well, the gynaecologist rabbited on about what they were going to remove, instead of answering my questions. I found it hard at first, as I expected to be told that I had a problem conceiving, not that I would never have another child and that I had cancer as well.

I was then referred to a gynaecologist in Cambridge who specialised in carcinoma of the female reproduction system and embarked on a round of appointments to establish to what extent it had spread. This particular gynaecologist was excellent, he did everything he could to enable me to have another child. I had a cone biopsy first to see if that would clear the cancerous cells as the MRI scan had not detected any cancerous areas. After the cone biopsy procedure the gynaecologist explained that it was not looking too hopeful as I had lost a lot of blood and the blood flow had not stopped quickly enough, which indicated that the cells had progressed further, but I had to wait until confirmation from Pathology.

I made the final decision and the Wertheims hysterectomy was performed a week later. Due to my age (31), I wanted to keep my ovaries, to try and prevent an early menopause and I also wanted the scar to be as low as possible.

Up to the day of the operation I felt as if it was all happening to someone else and I was looking on. I was petrified on the day of the operation, but it went well and I managed to leave hospital two days early. After a week at home, with help I started to get back to normal, but different relatives continued to help out for another five weeks until we moved house. I did intend to return to my part-time job, but after four months off I resigned and became a full-time mother.

Post-operative, I had no feeling in my right leg near the pubic area, but that returned within a year. I also had abdominal pain which was diagnosed as an ovarian cyst, possibly caused by the surgery. I returned to the gynaecologist in Cambridge, who checked me over, plus taking X-rays. There didn't appear to be anything suspicious, so it was a case of seeing whether it would settle down.

At present I have checks done every four months, but each year these will be increased by one month until there is only one check a year. I will probably opt to have a six-monthly check undertaken for life, so that if the cancer does return it will be found at an early stage and I would feel more confident if it was every six months.

I do worry when my check is due, and I am quite stressed until I receive the results. I do feel it is only natural to worry about "What happens if it returns?"

After something like this happens to you, it is bound to change you - I know I have changed, and I feel sure my husband would agree. I have always been a strong person, but now I try to be more assertive, and I will not put up with anything that makes me unhappy. I have reassessed my life and thought about what I want to achieve and hopefully 1998 will be the year when particular goals will come to fruition. I am returning to college to study for a new career, which I have wanted to do for some years.

"Life after cancer" - Delia and Adrian's story

After a 'slightly abnormal' smear and having a slight discharge and abnormal bleeding I was sent for a colposcopy. A week before the appointment, whilst on holiday in Cyprus, aged 27, my husband and I decided that maybe it was the right time to try for a baby.

I was certain the colposcopy was only routine. I went along with a healthy suntan and certainly showed no visual signs of a life-threatening disease. Before going in to be examined, the nurse told me that if the consultant found it necessary to take a biopsy, the results would take approximately three weeks.

The colposcopy itself was relatively painless, but I was immediately summoned to the consultant's office - "You have cervical cancer and you will never have children." He also said that he didn't want to wait three weeks for the official results as we had to start treatment immediately.

I will never forget his words. At the time I hated him, he seemed so cruel to sit there opposite me and turn my life upside-down - my plans for children dashed and my life in jeopardy. However, looking back, I am pleased he was honest and, although he was harsh, I can't imagine that kind of news to be pleasant in any form. Once we had decided the best treatment for me, he was always there, and even once he was in hospital himself, on a phone from his bed advising a colleague of my treatment. He is a great doctor for whom I have the utmost respect and even though I hated him on that day I am pleased he was, and still is, my consultant.

The words were unreal and didn't mean a thing - I felt numb. Within minutes I was having blood tests, chest X-rays and booking in for a CT scan. I felt sure someone, somewhere had made a terrible mistake -- I didn't feel ill!

It was particularly hard at the age of 27 to be told that I would never have children and that my life was at risk. This was especially hard on my husband who found it difficult to cope with. Two years after my treatment and when I appeared well, he felt he had to go back to a counsellor to deal with all that had happened. The whole thing lives with you every day and is on-going, it has changed our lives.

After a further visit to the hospital, and more tests, I was told that things were more serious and my chances were slim, my cancer was too advanced for surgery and had most definitely spread into my pelvic area and possibly my lymph nodes. On that day I was taken to a room, given a cup of tea and put through to a hospital counsellor on the phone who gave me the number of BACUP and suggested I contact them.

Being offered counselling, after more bad news, was too much to take in on that day and I wasn't really interested. I still felt it wasn't me they were all talking about, I looked and felt so 'normal'.

Later on, a visit from the hospital counsellor was appreciated as I had had time to think and come to terms with things more. Much later my GP offered my husband and me group stress counselling at our surgery which was very useful and helped us both.

A hysterectomy was not an option and my first treatment was to be by external radiotherapy for three weeks — 15 sessions. I went through the process of being 'measured up' for the radiation — in a dark room with lots of calculating machines and two very nice nurses.

The first few sessions of radiotherapy went well and I felt no side effects. I did feel a little tired and I was covered in 'arrows' drawn in over my legs and stomach linking to my three tattoo marks in my pelvic region. They decided to 'zap' a large area — my ovaries were destroyed in my first radiotherapy session.

As the days went on the treatment took its toll — how could two minutes of radiation daily make me feel so ill? By the end of the three weeks I couldn't make the 20 minute car journey without a sick bag and had to rush to the toilet as soon as I got there. I was given medication to help with the sickness and diarrhoea but I did lose a lot of weight. The nurses were worried that if I lost any more they wouldn't be able to align the tattoos and arrows with the red beam of radiation and the treatment would be invalid.

I did want to eat, I had an appetite, and I would have done anything for my bottom not to pass anything as it was so sore. I remember thinking "if I can ever eat properly again I will never diet!". My friends had a rota going and every day someone different would appear on my doorstep to take me to the hospital. It gave my husband a break and gave me the will to fight because everyone was on my side and they believed in me. The radiotherapy nurses were wonderful and always explained, and showed my friends, the fascinating and precise process that they went through for each patient. By this time, taking my trousers down and exposing my arrows and tattoos seemed natural - pubic hair was a thing of the past!

Every day I used to lie there during my treatment, and imagine an army on horseback fighting the tumour - and of course winning! I was given a week off to try and recover from the treatment, and then admitted to hospital for the next stage— internal radiotherapy. This was probably the worst time for me. I was in a room on my own, surrounded by lead screens, visitors were only allowed to stay for thirty minutes in any 24 hours.

After having had constant diarrhoea, I was now given strong medication for the reverse to happen. The rods (three in total) were put in under a general anaesthetic, with approximately one to two inches of the rods visible outside of my vagina. A catheter was put in at the same time. I wasn't allowed out of bed for five days and had to try and lay still so as not to move the rods out of position.

It was a very sad time for me with lots of time to think. I didn't see many people as the nurses were only allowed a limited time of access to the room to protect themselves from the radiation, and I think my friends were afraid of what they might see. It was at this time that my best friend's husband came to see me to break the news that his wife was pregnant and wasn't allowed to visit me. I found that hard as Adrian and I had always planned to have children together. I decided that I didn't want something so exciting for my friends to turn into a nightmare because of me, and felt that I had to be strong for all of us.

I had trouble with my catheter and kept wetting the bed, and so was scared to drink too much. And then was told off for not drinking enough as I would get an infection. I started to feel sores on my bottom and on my heels from staying in one position too long — how much in life we take for granted!

Five days later the rods were removed by two nurses, in my room. I was really scared about this as one of the nurses told me I had been in 'trauma' whilst trying to get the rods in as they couldn't get one of them over the tumour. I was given pethadine for the pain. I couldn't believe how much packing had been inside of me, and I actually recall likening it to a magician's hat (strange how the mind works at intense moments).I was then allowed home where the diarrhoea and vomiting returned. Once treatment had been completed and the side effects had settled down, I was recalled for a CT scan to see how I had responded to the treatment. I couldn't believe the news: "There is no sign of the tumour"!

I returned back to work three months after the first diagnosis. It was quite a big step as I am an air stewardess and have to look and feel good. It was my decision to go back as I had to have something to aim for. Sometimes everyday life is hard as my bowel was affected by the radiotherapy and so my toilet habits are now embarrassing and rather urgent at times! Also as a result of the treatment my whole reproductive system was destroyed and I became a menopausal woman aged 27.

I have been continually well over the last few years with only the odd bout of cystitis, and I have just been given the 'five year all clear'. Every day I think how lucky I am to be here and how precious life really is. My consultant can't believe how well I responded to the treatment. I put a lot of it down to sheer determination and the will to live, plus the support of a wonderful husband, family and friends. If I'm having a bad day, I read through all my cards and letters that I received at the time and it reminds me how good life is now. I feel I have a lot left to achieve and have no fear of anything. Since I recovered I've been skydiving, wing walking, white water rafting and lots more.

Cancer turned our lives upside down and made us re-evaluate our priorities, but we have come through as a much stronger and closer couple than anyone I know. We can't have children but that is a small price to pay for being alive, and we have enough nieces, nephews and godchildren to fill that gap. Life is great, and since cancer we have lived and worked in New Zealand and Germany and always look forward to our next adventure. Life is full of opportunities there for the taking. The whole thing lives with you everyday, and is on-going, it has changed our lives but there really is life after cancer!

Adrian's story - a husband's experience

It doesn't matter how close you feel you might be to your partner, because when they are told they have cancer you might as well be on another planet. At least, that is how I felt.

Delia was diagnosed in September 1992 and her prognosis was not good. I have tried to analyse my emotions many times since that day but like many men you tend to sweep them under the carpet, because that is what real men do - or is it?

Laying in bed looking at the ceiling became an occupational pastime. I couldn't get my head around the fact that there was nothing I could physically do to help. As a man it was always fairly easy. If anyone was attacking your wife, partner or children, you would protect them, but here I was trying to pick a fight with something I couldn't see.

Everyone tells you to expect anger, but in my mind the frustration was just as bad.

Meanwhile Delia was starting to fight her own personal battle. I began to realise that my own anger and frustration could be redirected to helping her by being supportive and strong, but most of all, normal. Delia was undergoing constant medical evaluation and treatment, but I realised that what she wanted was to escape to her normal environment. That was the thing that was going to help her form a base from which to fight.

The medical teams which we were dealing with in this case were excellent: encouraging me to provide the required level of normality. That was the easy part — I just carried on leaving the toilet seat up!

Delia responded to the treatment very well and her recovery is told above in her own words. After all the drama 'normal life' has to go on. This is the hard part because life can never be the same again, but then, why should it be? Nothing is more apparent from the experience than that life is so precious. Some of my friends can't understand our reluctance to play the lottery. All I say is: "Haven't we already won?!"

Living with somebody who has cancer is terrible, but for goodness-sake never feel isolated, never worry about an inability to express emotions, just be there. That is the best thing you can do.

Heather's story

I was deputy head of an infant school, with two children aged 10 and 6 at home, when diagnosed in 1991, aged 39. This was the first time I had actually stopped for as long as

I could remember. My thirties had been like a blur, working hard, going on courses, bringing up children, and I was also deeply unhappy in my marriage, which the 'busyness' of my life had masked, to a degree. Cancer changed the whole course of my life — it made me look at what I was doing and I realised that only I could change it. Six years on, my knowledge of complementary therapies and ways in which we can help ourselves has grown tremendously, but I work at keeping healthy and well all the time, it's an on-going process!

I qualified as a teacher in 1973 and, apart from two maternity leaves, I had taught infants constantly from then until my diagnosis. I was a conscientious teacher, and also the main breadwinner for many years while my husband was at college as a mature student.

During the year preceding the diagnosis, I had felt constantly unwell - tired, recurrent sinusitus, headaches, thrush, candida problems. I had been prescribed several courses of antibiotics for the sinusitis - none of which worked - and I eventually tried acupuncture. This did work, but the most important thing to me about this was that when I told the acupuncturist I felt as if I was on a treadmill and couldn't get off, he replied that I could, there were always ways of stopping and changing. My reply to that was a definite "No, I can't!"

Well, my body knew better, and two months after this, I noticed small spots of blood on the bedsheet occasionally — which I ignored because I was too busy to think about them. Then, after a smear test, I didn't stop bleeding and I knew there was something wrong.

I received the result of the test — severely abnormal — on Christmas Eve 1990, and was admitted for a cone biopsy on Valentine's Day 1991. Two weeks later I received the diagnosis of cancer by post. By accident I had been sent my first appointment at the oncology and radiotherapy department before I had seen the consultant who was to break the news to me. I was extremely shocked, and all I can remember of that evening is attending the retirement party of my school's secretary and feeling as if I was in a film.

I had decided to go back to school until I started the radiotherapy, but the following day my friend Maggie, who had had cancer three times, brought me a copy of *The Bristol Programme* by Penny Brohn (this book is now out of print, but may be available from libraries), one of the co-founders of the Bristol Cancer Help Centre. I read this non-stop that weekend and it completely changed my life. I never returned to school, I realised I could do so much to help myself to get better, and I resonate totally with the ideas in the book. I told my husband that I wasn't returning to work, I wanted to concentrate on getting well, I would make no definite plans on whether I would eventually return to work, but that if I did it would definitely be part-time. I had never been so assertive before!

My marriage was not happy but I attach no blame to anyone for this. My husband was dominant, but I allowed it to be so. I believed in marriage and wanted to make it work for the children's sake too, but in pleasing other people I neglected myself. Having cancer made me realise this: for the first time in my life I concentrated on myself.

I had a some time before the six weeks of radiotherapy started, and I used this period to learn to relax, to read positive and uplifting books, to learn to visualise, to seek out people and therapies that could help me, to start vitamin and nutritional strategies to begin the healing process. What I actually realised I was doing was nourishing myself. My husband was very caring and supportive at this time, and I enjoyed the attention. Obviously there were extremely bad moments of despair and despondency, especially early in the mornings, but I lived positively as much as I could.

I took arnica before beginning radiotherapy, and also all the vitamins recommended by the BCHC, but as the treatment progressed I couldn't bear to swallow tablets. I had radium rods inserted under general anaesthetic, twice, and daily external blasts of radiation, and by the end of the six weeks I felt terrible. I was nauseous, could only eat chocolate and potatoes, couldn't drink anything, had diarrhoea, piles, thrush, cystitis, aches all over, etc., etc. I couldn't sleep, couldn't do anything, and I had begun the menopause with hot flushes.

However, throughout that time I had persevered with the visualisation (so much so that the radiographers commented on how relaxed I was), the listening to tapes and reading books. I had healing each week and I discovered that having a session of zero-balancing actually lifted the effects of the radiation for an hour or so.

My visualisation had been of a cartoon white piranha fish eating black dots which were the cancer cells, and towards the end of the six weeks, I couldn't manufacture any black dots — the piranha fish were swimming around aimlessly. I felt intuitively that the cancer had gone, but not strong enough to say I wanted to stop the remaining radiation treatments!

Slowly I began to heal and to get better. Every day I relaxed, meditated, exercised, ate nourishing wholesome food, took the vitamins. I was so happy to be alive.

I took early retirement from teaching, and I have spent the last six years discovering myself, finding out the real me. Ultimately this has lead to the break up of my marriage, but I feel that now I am truly being me for the first time in my life.

I have read a lot about the nature of cancer, spent time at the BCHC, and I am convinced that it is an emotional disease. In my case, I had spent most of my life fearful, anxious, eager to please and to be liked, lacking in self-esteem and self-respect. I had an abortion at 30 because my husband was angry that I had become pregnant with the coil in and I agreed to it because I was afraid to say no — it went wrong and I had to have it done again three days later. I suffered with an infection afterwards, and a back problem.

At about this time my husband's sexual desires became more perverse, and although I hated it, I gave in to keep the peace, to keep everyone happy. I had no-one to confide in, I was working hard, I was distraught after the abortion, I had a two year-old child, and I looked serene on the outside. I held it all in: I had persistent thrush, I was tired, I was deeply unhappy, and I dreaded every weekend when I knew I would have to 'please' my husband. I felt there was no way out. There was, but I couldn't see it — I blamed myself for not wanting to do the same things sexually as my husband — I felt that there was something wrong with me.

Eventually I had my second child, which was lovely, but my pregnancy was tarnished by the sexual demands and deviations of my husband. Still I told no-one, held it all in, and this went on, getting worse and worse, all through my thirties, until I got cervical cancer.

I am absolutely convinced that I held deep emotions in my womb— guilt and sadness over the abortion, resentment towards my husband, and having read *Women's Bodies, Women's Wisdom*, [Ed: See reading list.] it has strengthened my conviction.

I feel strongly that in my own case, working too hard and for too long; holding unhappiness in; pretending to be serene when I was angry, resentful and fearful; not looking after my own inner needs; not feeling as if I was good enough, even when I was outwardly successful — were the most important factors in my cancer. I also feel that my body, at the end, was rejecting my husband. I ate a healthy diet and exercised — it was basically unhappiness over a long period.

Helen's story

Early in 1991, I was having problems with, as I thought at the time, heavy periods. These got progressively worse and longer over a very short period of time. I visited my GP to be seen by a locum and was told that I was probably going through an early menopause, and that unfortunately some women suffer more at this time than others. So, basically I thought that was it, and I had to put up with it, I was destined to have erratic and heavy periods till after I'd got through the menopause.

By September 1991, my periods were practically constant with only a day or two in-between if I was lucky. Worse still I would flood with no notice whatsoever and lose very large liver-like clots of blood. It became so bad that I was housebound most of the time, unable even to go over to visit a friend across the road. I used to sit on a chair with a plastic covering over the cushion and on top of a pile of bath towels — yes, it really was that bad, and yes, I really did believe what the locum had told me, and that this was my lot, and I had to tolerate it!

By the beginning of October I had had enough. The bleeding had continued with no let up, I was becoming increasingly tired and irritable which I put down to the excessive blood loss and the frustration of the whole absurd situation. When I had a day when I was virtually clear, (these were very few and far between) I telephoned my GP and after some pressurisation and insistence, managed to get an emergency appointment. I explained to my GP all that had been going on and he managed to take a cervical smear, but I began to bleed immediately. He said that he would refer me to a gynaecologist, but that the waiting list was fairly long, so I asked him to request an early appointment if a cancellation became available.

Less than a week later I received an appointment in the post to see a consultant at the hospital exactly seven days after I'd had the cervical smear. Naively, I assumed that this was a cancelled appointment — fortunately, though she did not say so at the time, my friend suspected that there may be more to it and insisted on accompanying me. All I was told at the time was that they had discovered some abnormal cells, and wanted to do a cone biopsy and D&C. I was told that the D&C should alleviate the horrendous bleeding that I'd been getting, and that the cone biopsy would probably clear the abnormal cells and enable them to be tested to see exactly what they were.

At this stage I was not unduly worried. In fact I was looking forward to the D&C, as the thought of being able to have days free from the bleeding was bliss.

My operation was successfully done two weeks later. I was told that I would be given a follow-up appointment about seven days after my discharge to be given my results. Five days after discharge I had a letter with an appointment from the Radiology Department at the hospital. I telephoned my consultant in a panic and he saw me the same day to give me the results which basically boiled down to the fact that I had a cancerous tumour on the cervix.

Fortunately, again my friend came with me, and asked some questions on my behalf that I was frankly in no fit state to even think about, let alone ask. I was asked at some point why I hadn't been to see my GP earlier, and I explained what had happened. I was also asked if I had consulted my GP about my tiredness, and I said no. I mean — if every woman who felt tired went to see their doctor they would have a full waiting room 24 hours a day, 365 days a year!

Initially I was in a state of shock. After hearing the word 'cancer' I did not hear anything else I was told — I just wrote myself off and buried myself in my mind. Unless you have been through a similar experience, nobody can begin to understand the complete desolation that sweeps over you, the fear, the worry, the guilt, the overwhelming anger, and a strange isolating feeling of being alone. The range of emotions is wide and I feel must be unique to people in this situation.

I spent the next few weeks up until Christmas as if I was in some sort of void. I went to the hospital for various appointments, but I couldn't tell you exactly what they were for. It was as if no matter what 'they' told me, I knew in my mind that was going to die. I never voiced my many fears to my family or to my friends, they all thought that I was coping remarkably well, and that I'd come to terms with the situation. Nothing could have been further from the truth! The constant fear and worry of the whole situation was escalating.

One of the greatest of these fears was what would become of my beloved daughters? My eldest daughter was seventeen at the time, with her whole life ahead of her. How could she be expected to cope and look after her two sisters who at the time were only four and five years old. This was too great a burden to be placing at her door. I didn't know what to do, but I kept my thoughts to myself, hoping that something could be sorted out when the time came.

I made my mind up to have a good Christmas, and try to make it as good as possible for my children. It was great, and normality almost returned for a few days when I managed to block out the inner madness which I felt was in danger of consuming me totally.

The respite was all too brief. The day after Boxing Day, I attended Churchill Hospital, Oxford, for my radiotherapy planning. I was given BACUP's telephone number to get some detailed information about cervical cancer and the radiotherapy treatment on which I was about to embark.

One week later, the day after New Year's Day, I started my radiotherapy treatment — 25 sessions with only weekends off — Happy New Year!! My treatment was fine to start with, but as time went on the side effects started to show. Now I understood why I was told — much to my distaste — that I was not to use any soap, bubble bath, personal deodorants, talcs, etc. The further I got into the treatment, the worse the side effects became, and towards the end of the treatment they were horrendous. Complete rawness of the skin — internally and as well as externally — so much so that it was unbearable to touch, and I had to be prescribed some strong pain-killers to get me through. Complete exhaustion, I could sleep anywhere, including on the sometimes rather uncomfortable transport provided to get me from where I live in Swindon to Oxford.

These were my two worst side effects, the rest I coped with very well. Once my treatment had finished, and it didn't come a day too soon, I was told that after I had had a chance to recover, I would have to return to have an internal source of radiotherapy. I was devastated — the thought of becoming relatively well again only to have further treatment, and an even more intensive treatment at that — was abhorrent to me. Although I was assured that the side effects would not be as severe, I didn't believe them considering that before the last treatment the same people had told that I might have a little soreness, feel a little tired — what an understatement that was!

About four weeks passed, and I was feeling a lot better, not a hundred percent, but OK. The dreaded day had arrived when I had to go back for the rest of my treatment. I was placed in a side room on my own behind a lead partition, the internal source was put in place and was to stay there for 28 hours. You had to lie still and in the same position for the whole time, not at all comfortable, but I tolerated it because I was told that if it was accidentally displaced the procedure would have to be done all over again.

Over the next few weeks I suddenly discovered that my attitude towards my cancer had changed. I can't say exactly when, only that it did. Although the fear was still very much there, a sort of acceptance of the situation and inner strength came over me. It is very hard to explain, but women who have been through this seem to understand exactly what I mean. I am convinced that much of it came from my experiences at Oxford, not from the treatment, but from the people that I met. These wonderful people of all ages who had a variety of different types of cancer, showed me courage, strength of character, compassion. empathy, caring, and strangely enough, humour. No matter what lay ahead I felt that I could at least face it with a little dignity.

At the end of May 1992 I had a radical hysterectomy. Everything was taken away - ovaries too. The operation was a success, and I recovered remarkably well. I expected it to be much worse than it actually was - yes, I did have some pain, but this was controlled by myself by means of PCA (Patient Controlled Analgesia). This enabled me to administer a measured dosage of morphine when it was required. It was removed after two days when conventional pain control was used. Perhaps I was fortunate, but I was up and about very quickly, and fared much better than some other women on the ward who had also had a hysterectomy (though they had had theirs for different reasons.) The experience of having had such a bad time during and after radiotherapy, and feeling so ill, made the hysterectomy seem like plain sailing.

I was prescribed HRT in patch form after this, but I did not get on too well with it, so I changed to tablets. I was told that it was best for me to have HRT as it would help to combat osteoporosis (brittle bone disease) in later life, and would also stave off any menopausal symptoms that I might experience due to the removal of my ovaries. They were a bit late with that as one of the effects of the radiotherapy was that it had already damaged my ovaries, and so I had been experiencing hot flushes and night sweats for some time. On discharge from the hospital, I felt fine. I was very fortunate in that I had very supportive friends and family who made sure that things like the housework and shopping were looked after.

Two days before my six week check-up at the hospital, my left leg swelled up like a balloon very quickly, so much so that I was unable to walk and was in great pain, it felt as if it would burst at any moment. I sent for the doctor who told me I had a lymphodema and gave me painkillers and water tablets to help reduce the swelling quickly. I managed to get to the check-up with great difficulty and in great pain — I had to get a taxi to the hospital and back. The check-up was with my consultant gynaecologist and the specialist in charge of my radiotherapy treatment. Afterwards I asked if the lymphodema had anything to do with my hysterectomy and was told that the lymph gland had probably been damaged by the radiotherapy treatment, and had been removed as a precautionary measure to ensure that the cancer had been contained. I was informed that this occurrence was very rare, but I have since found that it is fairly common for women who have had radiotherapy for a gynae cancer, particularly cervical cancer, to get lymphodema in one or other and occasionally both legs.

Apart from this, my consultant was pleased with me, and told me that I would have check-ups for five years, initially at three monthly intervals, stretching to annually at the end of this period. I was a little alarmed at this, but was more at ease once it was explained that this was normal procedure.

The lymphodema was really painful for some weeks, but the swelling did go down slightly. My GP said that "it would get better" and that I should "rest it" and "put my leg up". Well, I dutifully followed instructions for months with no great improvement. In the meantime my GP retired and I was assigned to a new doctor within the practice. When I visited him I was told that the condition would never get better, and that although I should take care, I could walk around etc. I was pleased that I could get around - but so angry at the mis-information from my old GP. Throughout the time I was with him I never had cause to complain and he was lovely, but I felt that rather than give me the facts he told me what I wanted to hear.

Anyway, more than five years down the line I am still here, still have lymphodema, still get very tired from time to time, do not sleep at all well. I have just one more appointment before being discharged from the hospital - in fact, I will probably have been by the time you read this. Despite the initial failure to refer me to the hospital and the mis-information over my leg, I am very grateful to all concerned for the speed and quality of the service I received, and to hospital staff for their kindness and attention. Although there is always room for improvement, I feel that they did the best that they could for me at that time, and I cannot thank them enough for that.

For anyone reading this who has had a similar experience, you will probably understand me when I say that my life has changed. I value each day as it comes, appreciate my family and friends much more than I ever did, and can now see the cushion of love and care with which they surrounded me during my treatment and beyond. This was particularly noticeable in my dearest dad, now sadly gone from this world, who used to drive almost daily a 32 mile round trip on any pretext just to make sure I was OK. I used to feel quite guilty about this as he wasn't a well man himself, but I now realise that it was something that he needed to do to reassure me that he and my mum were there for me, and to make sure that I really was on the mend.

Due to my experiences, and the fact that there wasn't a help-line or organisation available to contact at the time when I felt I needed one, I have started a self-help group called Gynae-C to offer confidential support and information to all women with any form of gynaecological cancer. I did a lot of background work prior to starting the group and discovered to my amazement that at the time there were no other groups dealing specifically with gynae cancer, and even now with the exception of Ovacome (dealing with ovarian cancer) there are virtually no other known groups or help-lines such as that of Gynae-C.

The help-line is used extensively by women from all over the UK, who are given our number by organisations such as CancerBACUP and Cancerlink. It is also available to partners, family and friends of the women involved. We receive an average of 25 calls per week, mainly from women newly diagnosed with a form of gynae cancer. These calls can range from a five minute time span to well over an hour. We do not have any set help-line times. The number is available 24 hours a day and when it is unmanned people can leave their name and number and we will always call them back. We are very discreet, so if the person is not available when we call back, we always give our Christian name as the caller and nothing else - not everybody wants anyone to know that they have contacted a help-line no matter how close they are. These are unique circumstances, and we can act as a sounding block for you to voice your fears without concerning your loved ones. Our help-line is operated by women who have had a gynae cancer themselves and so understand your worries and concerns. We offer empathetic emotional support at any time when it is needed, details of where you can get information from a quarterly newsletter, for which we invite letters and/or articles for inclusion (anonymously if you prefer). We welcome any further assistance e.g. if there is anyone willing to be a telephone contact/hold a local group meeting/organise a fund-raising event — anything is acceptable including raffles, sponsored events, car boot sales, fetes, bazaars, etc.

Please do not hesitate to ring us for the help-line or for details regarding any of the above, or write to us at:

Gynae-C, 1 Bolingbroke Road, Swindon, Wiltshire, SN2 2LB, Tel: 01793 480298, (contact details also listed in Appendix 2)

Jane's story

I started having abnormal smears in my late 20s, towards the end of the 1970s. For years I got results with mild abnormalities and was recalled after twelve months, or sometimes six months. This went on for about ten years, with constant mild abnormalities being found.

Then in 1987 or 1988 the level of abnormality suddenly jumped up a couple of notches (coinciding with a great deal of work stress). I was recalled after three months, and then the same thing again. After three consecutive 'serious' (what used to be called Grade III/IV) abnormal smears my GP said she thought she should refer me to a gynaecologist.

The appointment came through within a couple of months. I prepared myself, and went expecting to have to deal with a stereotypically awful male gynaecologist — and he was wonderful! I saw the consultant, he spent 40 minutes with me, discussed the whole process, answered my questions, treated me as an intelligent adult, got all the 'signals' right, did the internal exam very sensitively ... I was gobsmacked, and wrote to him afterwards to thank him.

I was referred for a diathermy to have the affected areas zapped, and that was done a few weeks later, as a day-stay patient. After three months, the next smear was back to Grade III/IV and so were the next two (at three month intervals). During this period the smears were being done at outpatients, rather than at my GP's surgery, which was very inconvenient and a dreadful waste of time. I also didn't know from one visit to the next who I would see. I had my fair share (and more!) of junior housemen doing their first gynae outpatients clinic, looking dreadfully embarrassed, being taught how to do smears, with me as a guinea pig. The nurses saved the day quite often. One junior got my cervix trapped in the speculum when he released it too soon.....!

Anyway, after these three abnormals, it was back to the consultant, who said he thought a cone biopsy was the next step. I'd been told that the diathermy "dealt with 95%" of cases, and that the cone biopsy "dealt with 95% of what was left". That appointment came in a couple of months, and I was in hospital for four days. I found this very unpleasant and distressing - the vaginal pack, being confined to bed because of risk of haemorrhage.

After three months I went back for a smear - more of the outpatients experience as above! Again Grade III/IV - and twice more at three month intervals - I was now "5% of 5%" - one in 400! Back to the consultant again: the discussion was about a hysterectomy. He wasn't pushing me, he said it was important but not urgent, and if I "wanted to start a family" they would "keep an eye on me". I replied that I was 39, I wasn't about to start a family, and I really wanted all the messing about and worry to be over. So we agreed on a hysterectomy conserving my ovaries.

I had to wait six months for the operation, and it was during that waiting period that I found myself a therapist, to deal with the feelings that were then surfacing.

I was treated very well during the hysterectomy — it was a small, old hospital (now gone — absorbed into a huge new shiny one) with a very good atmosphere. I was treated by the consultant and a female registrar, who did a good job in all ways. I went back for my six weeks post-op check-up, and then they didn't want to see me for twelve months. After a year I had an outpatients appointment for a vault smear, and went along feeling "this is it — now I'll be able to believe it's really all over."

Five days later, a small brown envelope, with the hospital district postmark, popped through the door, and I just stared at it with horror. The only reason they could be writing to me would be because there was something wrong. I opened it and there was just an appointment card, no letter, no explanation.

The following day I had a note from my GP, inviting me to talk it over with her if I wanted. She had been very good all along, discussing each stage with me, helping me sort out what questions I needed to ask the consultant. I talked with her, and saw the consultant a couple of weeks later. He was very good, and handled me and the situation, and my upsetness very well. He said he needed to refer me on to a regional facility for a colposcopy.

That took a couple of months to come through, and as I was now an 'interesting case', I saw the top specialist in the field - but had to go through the business of preparing to deal with a new consultant. He was mostly OK, though he lacked the warmth of my previous consultant. Also he mishandled bringing in someone else to look at me (in me, actually)— he didn't ask my permission beforehand. I found the colposcopy quite the most humiliating experience and I don't think anything could be done by anyone to make it better. The nurses fussed about and tried to distract me, which I found irritating.

He recommended laser treatment on the patch of affected vaginal skin - that was a day-stay op., about six weeks later, which he did himself. This hospital had not nearly such a pleasant atmosphere, and the anaesthetist was rude, patronising, bad-tempered. And I think I was given inadequate information about the aftermath of the laser treatment, I spent a lot of time phoning people, trying to find out.

I went back after three months and had another colposcopy, this time with the consultant plus a young female registrar. They found some over-granulated tissue in the wound and removed it, and that turned out to have some mildly abnormal cells in it.

But since then, all clear. I went back for two more colposcopies, at six month intervals, and was then referred back to my GP to have annual smears for a further six years. They have all been clear so far, and there is one more to go. If that remains clear, then it is back to every three years like everybody else.

In the post-hysterectomy phase I found it (and still do) extremely irritating when the nurse doing the paperwork just routinely asks "When was your last period?" — without bothering to glance at the notes. I understand why they do it, but I still find myself gritting my teeth when I say "September 1989!"

I think I was fortunate. It could have been a lot worse. The faults were mostly due to general NHS systems rather than particular individuals. Around the periods of surgery and anaesthetic I was also having acupuncture and homeopathy, just to help my body deal with the assaults it was suffering. In each case I recovered well and quickly.

Last thoughts: the biopsy they did after the hysterectomy showed fibroids, cervical erosion, and carcinoma in situ. They also told me I had polycystic ovaries. I did all my own info-finding about the hysterectomy - the system really told me very little. I expected to start menopause fairly soon after (two years is average apparently), but it seems to be happening now -- seven and a half years on, age 47— pretty normal age, really. Throughout the whole business, I've been acutely aware how an educated, intelligent, middle-class patient can get a better deal out of the NHS than people who don't fall into that category, and I played the game to my advantage.

"Bravery? No, I'm doing what I have to do." - Lisa's story

It began in September 1993. After a few months of what I thought were 'insignificant' bleeds (many post-coital), I began to experience a sharp pain in my abdomen. I paid a visit to my GP, who thought it was something or nothing. I began to put on weight, feel lethargic, and my periods became increasingly heavy and painful.

As I had not had a smear test for five or six years (now to my regret), my GP encouraged me to have one, which revealed abnormal cells. It shook me to hear this news, but I was aware that many women receive the same results and go on to find out that they are absolutely fine. Therefore, although I was concerned about the symptoms, I wasn't too worried. Three months later I underwent a colposcopy investigation. By then I was very tense and nervous anyway, but the look on my gynaecologist's face sent a wave of fear through me. So when, a few days later, I entered hospital for a cone biopsy, part of me knew that there was something very seriously wrong. A few days later, when I was told that

I had a malignant tumour on my cervix, I was shocked to say the least. You never expect to be told that you have cancer (though the word 'cancer' was never mentioned!).

I was only 24 when I was diagnosed, alone, raising a five year old daughter. Like anyone diagnosed with cancer, I was terrified, angry, shocked, etc., etc. After a rather probing and distressing consultation with a house doctor a few weeks later I felt that I was just left to face the fear and confusion of this illness alone. Having to wait three months to have a hysterectomy, I still believe was ridiculous. No counselling was offered, though my surgeon was wonderful and made personal telephone calls to myself and my mother to reassure us.

In August 1994, I entered hospital for a radical hysterectomy - it was a nightmare. An hour before the surgery I had a blood transfusion, the surgery lasted five and a half hours, followed by another transfusion. During the following week my spirits began to lift, relieved that it was all over, only to be told, the day I left hospital, that the cancer had spread to my pelvic lymph glands. An MRI scan two months earlier did not reveal this — maybe the time spent waiting for the operation had allowed the cancer to spread? I'll never know.

Six weeks later, radiotherapy began. The sickness and other symptoms would have been bearable if I hadn't had to spend five days a week having treatment 100 miles away from my daughter. After the internal radiotherapy, my spirits were at an all-time low, but within weeks life started to seem brighter. I began a part-time job, my social life improved, and everything got back to 'normal'.

Ten months after my radiotherapy treatment finished, a scan revealed that the cancer had returned in my lymph glands. The news hit me harder than the original diagnosis, particularly when I discovered that the cancer, though treatable, is now incurable. I was offered six treatments of chemotherapy. After three, a scan showed the tumours had dissolved, but after four, physically, and especially emotionally, I felt I couldn't take any more, and ended treatment.

That was nearly two years ago now, and the cancer has held off and I feel great. I feel very positive, and physically, I feel almost as if my body hasn't been through the torture that it has. I still have some pain in my abdomen and for a long time was reluctant to have any sort of intimacy again (whether emotional or physical). Also I am still trying to deal with the way my body looks due to surgery. However, over the last year I have begun to develop relationships again, which has given me much more self-confidence. Also I am learning to drive — I never had the courage before — and planning a holiday abroad with my daughter.

The only regret I have is being ignorant to the fact that regular smear tests were important even for someone of 24 years, and that I was not aware of the significance of other symptoms. It would be useful also for more information to be available to inform people of services available to them. For example, I only recently found out that I could have a health visitor, and she has been very supportive. BACUP, Macmillan nurses, and the local hospice have all helped me in different ways. Since I was told of the recurrence it has been very difficult to cope emotionally, at times life has seemed unbearable. The Macmillan service were also able to help out financially, as I had to leave my part-time job when the cancer recurred, and things were very difficult.

However, for the first time since the cancer returned, I am enjoying life again. Cancer has made me a much fuller person, and although it has put me, my daughter and my family through hell at times, at least I can appreciate life and make the best of it. My daughter's love is my greatest weapon to fight the illness and my greatest strength.

Cancer doesn't have to be the end of your life. It could just be the start!

Tumour Humour! - Maggie's story

I'm calling my chapter 'Tumour Humour' to signify the type of grim humour that's helped me through the soul-searching, pain, distress and anger I have experienced in my long fight against cancer.

I was first diagnosed with cervical cancer in 1973, when I was 27. I had suffered months of mis-diagnosis: I'd been bleeding heavily, particularly during sex, for about eight months – and been told by various GPs that I had irregular periods, infections etc.

Eventually, sick of it all, I presented myself late one night at casualty, and was admitted immediately. After an emergency D&C, I was told by a consultant (with my first husband present) that "You have something growing inside you which, if it isn't treated, will become very bad." I went into immediate shock. The consultant dished out, on the spot, doses of valium, and advised me to keep taking them.

Maybe things have changed since then, but I needed time to sit, think, then return to the room to ask more questions — and have explanations given in plain English. There should be no immediate offers of anti-depressants — I became addicted to them. I had no NHS support, counselling, aftercare — nothing.

Also, two weeks prior to the diagnosis, I had had a clear smear. I feel that it is rarely stressed in articles and other advice that women should be aware of other symptoms — discharge, discomfort, bleeding — even if smears prove to be clear.

I was given radium implants and then a Wertheim's hysterectomy followed by six weeks of radiotherapy. My GP was so embarrassed about his ineptitude (I suspect he had been hauled over the coals by the surgeon) that he was waiting for me to come round from the anaesthetic. He apologised and said that he hadn't thought of suspecting cancer in one so young.

In those days no one spoke of cancer, hysterectomy, menopause — particularly to someone of my age. Some of the comments that were made to me seem unbelievable now. Three days after my operation, when I experienced my first 'hot flush', I told the consultant, and he said "Well, you expected that didn't you?" — I hadn't, I didn't know what a menopause was!!

When I complained that my hair was falling out, he snapped, "You're moaning about your hair, when you're lucky to be alive!" I remained in a valium-induced, menopausal blur for four years (I put on four stones), and in 1977 my husband left me — I was crazy, fat, and didn't understand what had happened to me.

I pulled through anyway, until, in 1983, following my annual colposcopy check-up, I received a phone call at 10.30pm one Sunday night (I was drunk at the time!) from the surgeon. He told me to come in the next day as irregular cells had been found, and I was admitted immediately for laser treatment.

After three months I attended for another colposcopy follow-up, and was told to ring three weeks later for the result — I was given the all-clear, over the phone, by the consultant's secretary. One week later, for my follow-up appointment, I bounced into the consultant's office — and was told that the secretary hadn't looked at both sets of results. In fact, I had cancer again, and a small part of my vagina would have to be removed. In floods of tears, I was left to drive home alone. I had the operation done a week later.

Another three months passed, another follow-up appointment, and cancer was diagnosed again. This time I had to have a substantial piece of vagina removed, which would make normal intercourse impossible. Distressed, I felt that my femaleness was under attack, so I said that I didn't want the operation unless an attempt was made, at the same time, to rebuild a false vagina. At this point, the consultant uttered the immortal words: "Why are you so concerned about intercourse at a time like this? Would you describe yourself as highly sexed?" (A question which still makes me feel as if I would like to kill him!).

At this point I decided that this man was not the man for me! I sought out another consultant in Oxford (I lived in Bristol at the time) who was skilled not only in removal of tumours, but also in vagina-plasty (rebuilding of vaginas for women who are born without them). I paid privately to see him, much to the disgust of the Bristol consultant, who said, "I could be doing this for you — why do you need to see him?"

I had to have my lymph system tested to see if there were any suspect cells, the consultant doing this said: "..if we find any there won't be any point in you going to Oxford will there...?", meaning: "..because you'll die!!" While she was doing the test she asked me what I would do if she found anything. I replied that I would get all my money out of the bank and go to Israel (my favourite place at the time). She said something to the effect that: "You needn't think you'll do that because you'll feel iller and iller, then weaker and weaker, you'll bleed more and more, and then your tumour will start to smell." These comments look unbelievable when written on paper, it seems as if they really wanted me to die for daring to switch to the consultant in Oxford.

I did have the tumour removed in Oxford, but the consultant was unable to rebuild my vagina because the tumour was so large, and proved very difficult to remove. When I returned to Bristol for my follow-up the consultant said, "I'm secretly glad you went to Oxford because I don't think I could have done it so well."

Six months later I returned to Oxford for a second attempt at vagina-plasty, but it failed, and in the attempt the surgeon spotted that the walls of my bladder and bowel were fused together as a result of radiotherapy, and that the walls of both were paper-thin. He also managed to puncture my bladder which meant that I was threatened with a urostomy bag, but after three weeks of lying prone in my hospital bed, the hole healed itself. After this he performed an episiotomy which now gives me some extra length of 'vagina'.

Three months later, more suspicious cells were found - this time I decided that I'd better do something myself. I went to the Bristol Cancer Help Centre, and with their help I radically altered my diet, embarked on vitamin and mineral therapy, visualisation, relaxation, and healing. Also - most importantly for me - psychotherapy, during which I uncovered buried grief about an abortion and my mother's death.

I got well — and it was hard. I'm never going to be one of those crazy people who writes, "I'm glad I got cancer - it made me strong." Cancer was, and is, awful. It was long, hard, disfiguring, weakening and a total bore and turn-off.

I'm still well, I use orthodox medicine for check-ups and tests, but I don't think I would submit myself to them again — I don't trust them, and I don't feel cared-for or healed by them. I have recently become a Reiki healer, and the healing that I underwent during my initiation has at last removed the damage done by radiotherapy after 22 years.

"God's tap on the shoulder" - Mary's story

The day I was told I had cancer is etched into my memory. I had already had an abnormal smear test, followed by a colposcopy examination and loop diathermy treatment (after a wait of six weeks) which had been extremely painful. I was in bed at home recovering from this when the telephone rang. It was the receptionist from my doctor's surgery asking me if I could come in to see her immediately. That feeling of shock, horror, dismay is described in clichés as 'my heart sank' — but is so much more terrible than that. When I started the car, literally shaking, the radio news came on with an announcement that John Smith, leader of the Labour Party, had died that morning — it added to the feeling of a portentous, doom-laden day.

When I arrived at the surgery I had to sit in the waiting room and even though there was no one else there, the piped music was still playing. It seemed so incongruous and intrusive, jingly-jangling through my head. The doctor broke the news as gently as she could, saying that she had just received a call from the doctor at the colposcopy clinic, and that I had cancer (I think she used the word - but I can't remember). A hysterectomy operation had already been booked for ten days later, though the consultant gynaecologist was on holiday so I wouldn't be able to see her until the Friday just before the operation. I was told I may need to have radiotherapy following the surgery.

All I could think of was I couldn't possibly take time off work, I had a job to do and I was needed there. I was also looking forward to attending a conference that my boss had funded me to attend, this was only five weeks after the date of the operation but the doctor encouraged me to think I would probably still be able to go, "it will be something to aim for." After I had finished gabbling about all these things I sat and looked at her as the real significance began at last to dawn on me: "Can I speak to someone else who has been through this?" She said she could not give me anyone's name because of patient confidentiality (though I have since learned that some doctors and consultants keep lists of volunteers prepared to talk and visit women who have just been diagnosed.)

As I left the surgery, shaking and in tears, the 'why me?' questions began to race through my head. I had been feeling unwell and stressed for some time. In fact the day in March that I was told I had an abnormal smear I had been to see the doctor to ask her what treatment she could advise to cope with stress. She had then promised to refer me to the community psychiatric nurse for counselling — but she had forgotten to do this.

During the six weeks after this before my appointment at the colposcopy clinic for loop diathermy, I don't remember being particularly worried about it, a colleague at work told me she had had a colposcopy and "it was nothing". Even at the clinic they only told me to take the afternoon off and not to lift anything heavy for a while. So I had returned to work the next day, a Friday, but had left early as the pain was so bad I couldn't work. The same had happened the following Monday — so I had returned to the doctor who had given me antibiotics in case I had an infection.

On that day in May, once I got home, I didn't cry, I phoned my husband at work, he understandably couldn't say anything adequate on the phone. Then I called my manager at the office, I remember saying: "Are you busy? I've got something rather important to tell you." I was still worrying about work — I was intending to go to work the next day, but she insisted I should not go in till the following Monday. I couldn't tell my mother on the telephone, I went there with my husband to break the news. I just felt guilty for the obvious shock on her face when she realised that it was cancer — I could hear myself being jolly and practical, saying it was one of the most treatable cancers, I had very good prospects, it had been caught early, etc.

On the doorstep when we got home was a big bouquet of flowers and a card from the staff at the office. Surprisingly perhaps, they did make me feel better — though I also realised this was the beginning of being treated as 'a cancer patient' not as just Mary any more. It was a long time before I was to lose that feeling. I sat down when I got home and wrote to my sister in New Zealand — I just could not break the news on the phone. I can't remember which friends I telephoned that night or in the days following — it was so difficult every time: "Hi, how are you?" they would say brightly, and I would have to say "Well actually....". I didn't manage to phone everyone I should have, after a while I just couldn't face another stunned silence.

I can't remember now how I heard about CancerBACUP, but it was in the first few days after my diagnosis. They sent me leaflets, and answered as many questions as they could. And didn't answer some, I asked one nurse about the survival statistics for cervical cancer: "Well, we don't use statistics", she said in her lovely soft voice, "everyone's particular illness is different so they are meaningless." Very good advice, and so tactfully phrased that I didn't worry too much about what the statistics might say (apparently or otherwise).

I do not remember what my husband and I talked about in those evenings leading up to the operation, most of the time I just literally cried on his shoulder, especially in the dark at night when I had spent all day trying to be cheerful and positive. Everyone's attitude to me was so strange, I felt as if I had left my old familiar world for ever. The future was dark, frightening, and, worst of all, unknown. Some days I would wake feeling fine, with the sun shining outside, then I would remember my situation and the black cloud would descend on me again.

Daily life was also very strange in that week before I was admitted to hospital. I attended a training day I had booked for myself: "Women in Management" or some such title. I had hoped that I would be able to forget my problems but I felt so removed from it all, and found it hard to act 'normally'. It was quite a long drive home, and I felt exhausted when I arrived, my face looked so grey and drawn that my husband had a shock when he saw me.

On the day before I went to hospital we had lunch with friends at a favourite pub. I felt like someone about to go into prison for a life sentence, or an astronaut about to leave for a voyage to a far-off planet, not knowing if I would ever be the same again, or even be alive in a year's time.

My mother drove me to the hospital and I had to make my way to the X-ray department before going to the gynae ward to be admitted. After having details taken by what seemed like all and sundry, I was given a bed, and told to make myself 'comfortable'. The consultant arrived on her rounds — she said: "You look like you are ready to go home!", apparently thinking she had already operated on me. The sister quickly corrected her, and she apologised, but I felt rather worried by this, thinking of the stories of mix-ups in hospitals. After a while I decided that I needed to go for a walk in the fresh air while I could, I wandered round the gardens outside, wishing I could run away and hide, perhaps I would wake up and find it had all been a dream.

Once back on the ward, the preparations began, antiseptic bath, shave, etc., before trying to get some sleep. I was glad my operation was scheduled for 9 a.m., at least I wouldn't have to wait too long. That morning, the last thing I remembered seeing was the face of the anaesthetist in his mask. Waking up after a general anaesthetic is terrible whatever the operation you have undergone. I was in dreadful pain, but the nurses made me as comfortable as possible. My husband had been phoning to find out if he could visit that evening. The first time I was not back from the theatre (the operation must have been about five hours), the second time, the nurse advised that I would be better having an injection to knock me out to get some rest from the pain. My poor husband was terribly worried, I know how would I have felt if it had been me sitting at home by myself, cuddling the cat for company, waiting for news.

During that first night after my operation I dreamt that my mother was at my bedside singing 'I had a little nut-tree', a favourite lullaby she sang to me many times when I was ill as a child. It was enormously comforting. When she visited for the first time, the following day, she said she had been sending "lots of loving thoughts". I told her of the dream, she hadn't been thinking about singing to me, how strange, but lovely, for that to be the way in which her thoughts came to me.

Regular visitors came after that — my mother and my husband, then my brother and his wife and baby son, various friends. Lots of cards and flowers. The other women in the ward were a great help, all sympathising and cheering each other up. I was the only one who had had a Wertheim's hysterectomy though, so it was a little depressing when the others seemed to be improving much more quickly than me. This wasn't really surprising as a Wertheim's hysterectomy involves the removal of the womb, ovaries, and part of the vagina as well as the associated lymph glands. A lot of cutting and dissection has to done internally to achieve this, therefore there is a lot more healing to happen afterwards than in an operation where only the womb is removed.

People came and went, I was moved away from the nurses' station to a small room off the ward, much quieter at night. There was a Bank Holiday weekend approaching and the ward was emptying. I had to have a catheter in for 8 days, which I found very uncomfortable. After the first couple of days I felt quite a bit better but then I seemed to be on a 'rollercoaster', my emotions up and down like mad.

I had terrible trouble with constipation, caused by the drugs given for pain. Someone suggested that trying to open your bowels was "like giving birth to nations", which made me smile when struggling on the loo. I was on huge doses of pain-killers, but I would wake myself up thrashing about in pain and very frightened. One wonderful nurse spent ages with me talking and comforting me. Due to the Bank Holiday there was a delay in processing the tests carried out on the tissue removed during the operation, so I was kept in suspense waiting to find out if the cancer had spread and I would require radiotherapy.

I had several conversations with a German junior doctor. She had recently moved here from her home country. We talked about her family, about the differences between our countries and our common experience of working in Australia — it was wonderful being treated as a person instead of a patient.

When my results finally came through, I heard the German doctor running along the corridor to my room — she had a look of real joy on her face as she told me all was clear. I felt great euphoria at the news, telephoned my husband and my mother, almost felt like jumping with joy (but it was too painful!).

But after a while the pain was bad again, and I made myself feel more miserable by thinking how ungrateful I was crying when I now had nothing to worry about. When you are in the middle of an emotional whirlwind, not to mentioned the hormonal mix-up in your body after having suddenly had all the 'working bits' removed, it is no wonder that unexplained weeping fits creep up on you. But when you are in the middle of it you don't realise that is why you feel so tearful, making the pain and discomfort even more hard to bear. In ways that I still do not really understand, I almost felt as if I was a fraud of some sort for feeling devastated by having cancer, when I was treated in a 'normal' gynaecological ward, and was told ten days following my operation that all the cancer had been removed.

I read afterwards that 'third-day depression' is a common post-operative occurrence, the patient feels much better after recovering from the immediate after-effects of the anaesthetic and operation, but then gets knocked back with a swing in emotions the opposite way. I felt a little aggrieved as patients of a different consultant in the same ward had different pain-control measures, and a nurse talking to them undertaking some sort of study (I never did find out what it was about exactly), I felt quite left out.

I had taken several of my favourite children's books with me to read, I found *The Hobbit* and *The Secret Garden* very comforting. I also wrote a lot of my thoughts and feelings in the diary that I had begun the day I was diagnosed.

The day I left hospital was strange — I had been looking forward to it intensely, but also felt worried about whether I would be able to cope at home on my own. The journey home was painful, I hadn't realised how bumpy the roads were! My husband had been working hard in the garden and prepared lots of surprises — hanging baskets full of flowers that I could see through the windows from my armchair, a fountain in our goldfish pond, a beautiful copper beech tree in a pot on the lawn. I was so overwhelmed that I cried.

That first night at home I got up at 2.45 a.m. as I was keeping my husband awake tossing with the pain. I wrapped myself in blankets and settled down in two armchairs. Later I phoned my sister in New Zealand, it was lovely to hear her voice, but the line was not very clear so it was hard to have a real conversation.

The summer of 1994 was a beautiful one, so I was able to spend a lot of time in the garden. In some ways it was a restful time, and I was able to enjoy the warm weather and the peace and tranquillity. My husband and my mother looked after me well, and a few friends came to visit. After a while, people began to expect me to be better, especially as I acquired a suntan, making me look much healthier than I felt.

I was still taking a lot of pain killers. I hoped to drive to my six week check up but I wasn't able to do this. I tried a few short trips, but they always ended in tears of pain and frustration.

I began working from home immediately after my check-up — part-time at first, as I still needed to sleep in the afternoons. At one stage the doctor prescribed anti-depressants, but I hated the way they made me feel — woozy and not in control, and I stopped taking them after a while.

Towards the end of October I went back to the office full-time, but I still needed maximum doses of pain-killers to keep going. I went back to the consultant for help and she referred me to the local physiotherapy department for a course of 'Curapulse' treatment. This is done using a machine to provide deep heat treatment to the area of the pain to promote healing. I was warned that it would initially make the pain worse, but was not prepared for how much worse it would be! Sometimes my husband was able to drive me to the hospital, but at other times I had to drive there myself before work, then drive to the office, which was in the opposite direction to the hospital — I would be in agony before I started my day's work.

At this time the company were starting an important new project with tight deadlines, and I was involved in managing the team working on this. I would arrive home every evening in tears, in too much pain to eat, or do anything. Eventually, the day after my birthday on 3rd November, the morning came when I just could not face any more — I rang the office to say I would be late in, and one of my colleagues made me realise I couldn't go on like this. She spoke to my boss, who said he had not realised that I was still in so much pain. He called me and said I should go on sick-leave and concentrate on getting better. I realise now that I was foolish to let the pressure build up again as it had before my diagnosis, but everyone — family, work, doctors, and myself — all expected me to be fit after three months, (and this was five months after my operation), so I tried to convince myself I was, even though the fact that I needed so many pain-killers should have made it obvious that I wasn't!

In spite of the worry of being on sick-pay (previously the company had paid my salary throughout my treatment, which was wonderful, especially for a small company with limited resources, but of course this had added to the pressure I felt to get back to work) — I felt hugely relieved at being able to relax and look after myself. I tried a few more Curapulse treatments, but could not take any more after a while, and it did not seem to help. I spoke to an independent physiotherapist (recommended by the local person in the Hysterectomy Network) who told me she would not advise carrying on with it if it caused so much pain.

I decided to try acupuncture — and a friend recommended a practitioner very close to my home, who is also a qualified doctor, which gave me confidence that the treatment would not cause any harm. The first consultation took nearly two hours. As he explained, one of the reasons why he prefers practising as an acupuncturist to working in the NHS is having time to spend with each patient. It was wonderful having someone to actually listen to all my problems. I found the acupuncture a little painful at times, but it helped me get off the pain-killers. I also slept a lot, read books, concentrated on getting well. I realise now that I should have not have tried to do so much so soon, just because the average recovery time from a hysterectomy was quoted as three months, this did not mean that I should ignore the signals that I needed more rest and time to recuperate.

After four weeks I began working again, mainly from home. I had arranged to install a home office, so I would have room for a computer to be able to work properly. Eventually a routine was established of two days in the main office and three days at home each week, which is still my normal working pattern and works very well.

About 14 months following my hysterectomy, after a lot of requests and a visit to another consultant, I was referred to a Pain Clinic. I was very pleased at this as I thought at last someone was taking my problems seriously. I had a very bad journey there (the hospital is about 60 miles from my home) — my car broke down so I had to call in on my husband at work and borrow his. It was a very wet day and there was a lot of traffic on the roads. When I finally arrived at the hospital I had trouble finding a parking space. Eventually I found my way upstairs to the clinic where I had to wait for an hour before I was called into another waiting area and given a questionnaire to fill in. This is apparently used to assess the patient's psychological state — but I am sure I would have given very different answers if I had filled it in quietly at home!

The doctor seemed very nice and we talked about the background to my pain problem in some detail. He also went through things that could affect the perception of pain, especially emotional factors. Eventually, he said that there was one thing he could try, to establish if a nerve-blocking treatment would help me. This was to inject some local anaesthetic into the area where the pain was worst — the theory being that if this removed the pain it showed that it was localised in that one place. This was excruciatingly painful and I ended up crying uncontrollably. I was comforted by a nurse with cups of tea and kind words, and eventually shown back into the consultant's room again.

Maybe the tears were as much a release of all the tension and worry I had been feeling as a reaction to the actual pain caused by the injection, but the consultant appeared to have made up his mind that basically there was nothing wrong with me. He said I should try talking to my women friends more. "When my wife has a problem she goes to lunch with her friends and it all gets sorted out." Suffice to say, I wasn't very impressed at this. I was very upset, and felt I was being labelled a nuisance, but decided to try and deal with my problems without the help of doctors for a while. I have learnt a lot more about relaxation techniques and visualisation, and read many books which have helped me. I have reflexology, massage and acupuncture occasionally which help in reducing the pain. Even though I do understand that a wide number of factors are at work in the way we feel pain at any particular time, I still feel that my pain came first and that my depression, tears etc., followed from this. I read a slogan somewhere: "If the patient says it hurts, it HURTS!", and another "Pain is whatever the person says it is."

I still have to be careful what I do, a 'spiral' of pain seems to build up if I overdo things. For example, following severe winter storms my telephone is still cut off as I write this (January 1998), and I have had to travel to work in the main office every day. I have been shocked and rather upset by how quickly my pain level has built up again, and it takes quite a considerable time for it to return to 'normal'. At least I do know that I can control it if I can stick to my routine, but it does take a long time to settle down again.

When things are bad it is hard to remember that chronic pain does not mean that something is wrong, (as acute pain does), and if you start worrying it makes the pain worse. It appears the pain must be caused by adhesions and/or scar tissue, which may heal gradually, or may continue to give trouble. It is possible that a laparoscopy to investigate and free any adhesions may help, but this involves the risks of a general anaesthetic and may not improve the situation at all, so I have not as yet decided to undergo this procedure.

It is hard for other people to appreciate that I can still be in pain after all this time. While trying to do my job well and be as normal as possible it is hard to then have to make it clear when I am having difficulty. It is easy to struggle on for too long for fear of letting people down, and being afraid of appearing to be continually complaining.

Nearly four years have now passed. In that time I have completed an MA in Education with the Open University (I was in the last year when diagnosed). I have also continued working full-time, making my enamel jewellery, developed my writing skills, met many new and inspiring people.

It takes a long time to come to terms with having had cancer, with all the emotions such a diagnosis raises. In the bustle of daily life and work it is easy to slip back into old habits, but I try to keep in mind the lessons I have learned about what is really important to me. A sense of wonder and joy at the small treasures of life, a sunny morning, a cosy winter evening, bird song, wild flowers, the surf breaking on the Cornish coast. And most of all the love of family and friends. These are the important things in life, as long as we have these and appreciate them we are rich beyond measure. As the saying goes, may be it does take 'God's tap on the shoulder', by way of a major illness, to make us realise this.

When things begin to get too much, I try to remember the serenity prayer:

God grant me the serenity to accept the things I cannot change,

the courage to change the things that I can,

and the wisdom to know the difference.

(Reinhold Niebuhr)

Nicola's Story

I am 33 years old and three years ago had a radical hysterectomy for cervical cancer. I had a ten-month old daughter and a busy computing career when I was diagnosed.

The discovery of the tumour was delayed — at my six-week post-natal check-up, a 'polyp' was found. I waited ten months to have this polyp removed on the NHS, by which time it was found to be a tumour. I never had any ill-feeling about this — just one of those things. The most bizarre thing had been a fully clear cervical smear a year earlier (it was double-checked after my diagnosis, but gave the same result). So if I hadn't given birth when I did, I almost certainly wouldn't be here now.

At the time, a friend of mine also had more advanced cervical cancer. She had two operations and both radio- and chemotherapy, but sadly died. When I spoke to her about my desire to throw in my computing career, she suggested I do like her and take up childminding. I did, and it was a great irony that I went on to care for her two primary school children after school, following her death, and became very close to them.

I was always quite philosophical about my cancer (but frightened to death, too, at times) and found it an almost enriching process, even when my prognosis was unknown. I now help run a small cancer support group and talk openly about my experiences to anyone who will listen, in the hope that more people (a) realise cancer can hit anyone at any time (b) will attend regular cervical screening.

I have been surprised at how the effects of my experience, both physical and psychological, have lingered for far longer than I would have anticipated. Basically I know I will never be the same again, physically, even though I only had a stage one tumour, and surgery which cured me. The physical problems I have now are:

Exhaustion. This was very bad for about 18 months. I would be tired all the time, and need to sleep in the afternoons, but it would increase dramatically at certain times. I remember so many times when I would suddenly and desperately want to lie down — on the floor of the supermarket, or wherever - and go to sleep, unable to take another step or think straight. I still tire very easily after physical exertion or stress. Driving has become extremely tiring, as has mental concentration (meetings and interviews).

Bowel difficulties. Dreadful constipation — up to three weeks between 'goes', and the 'going' only as a result of tablets or extra fibre. General loss of appetite and nausea as a result, at times when the constipation is bad. This has improved somewhat in the last three years but will probably always be with me. (The bowel hates to be handled during the surgery, and my surgeon had a really good feel to see if the cancer had spread). And my husband says flatulence, too.... I suppose he's probably right!

Bladder difficulties. This has been hard and is difficult to talk about. But I find it quite a strain (not painful, but difficult) to pass urine. Worse though — for the first 18 months or so I had a bizarre kind of incontinence. It wasn't like stress incontinence (when you lose a little urine after a cough, sneeze or exertion) — it was a sudden, total voiding of the bladder with literally only about two seconds' warning. It happened three times in public, much more often at home. It is particularly odd because I can usually go many hours with a full bladder, and relieve myself when I choose. Other times (happily, rarely now), I can have only had a cup of tea all day, and it will still happen. I think this is due to nerve damage around the bladder due to surgery, but I can't explain why the pattern is so erratic. I'm told there is little that can be done.

Numbness. The extensive surgery meant cutting through nerve trunks. These heal very slowly and left me with no feeling in my groin and down the first three-quarters of my front thighs. As the months passed, the numbness receded slowly up my legs and is now limited to the groin area, and is not too bad. I hope it will go completely. The numbness was unpleasant — the flesh felt dead and heavy.

Fluid retention. Again, this is slowly getting better but was quite bad for the first 18 months. Generally, a spongy abdomen below the waist, extending over the groin areas and into my upper front thighs. Added to the skin numbness, this was quite an unpleasant feeling. I believe this is due to the fact that my thorough surgeon removed 48 pairs of lymph nodes from my abdomen (it seems an awful lot but I'm sure I remember right) to check for metastasis, which means that fluids now don't drain away so well. I can't prove the relationship, but it seems to have contributed to the worsening of my cellulite — the fronts of my thighs look very loose and wobbly, although I am underweight for my height.

Loss of libido. I'm sure this is a problem for many women. I've found it difficult to cope with and of course it has had an effect, of sorts, on my marriage. I am still able to enjoy sex as much as ever — I just can't get aroused at all beforehand, so I'm almost never the instigator. Add to this the general level of tiredness, and you get the picture for my poor husband!

These are all small prices to pay in order to be with my family and see my daughter grow. I can't imagine what it would have been like to have other forms of therapy on top of all this, or to have had anything less than one of the top specialists in the field, thanks to the private health insurance I had through work.

Emotionally, my experiences have been mixed. I was told of my diagnosis at mid-day and by bed-time I can honestly say I had come to terms with the possibility of my own death (no-one at that early stage could say what my prognosis was, so of course I assumed the worst). My Christian faith was strong, I had a loving family, had had a child, had lived 'enough'. That's not to say that I wasn't afraid, just that I could face it. I never asked 'why me'. Why anyone? Why not me? I was never angry for the first year. Anger came later, through other people's insensitivity. Or seeing how other people managed to plan their lives (like when to have their children, to fit in with holidays etc.) and how things worked out for them perfectly. But on the whole there hasn't been much anger, and no bitterness. Death is part of life and it has been helpful to face it, even if I have since been able to put the idea aside for a while.

My husband was hopelessly optimistic throughout my treatment — as his own defence mechanism, I suppose. He was always by my side but wouldn't talk about what might happen. This left me feeling frustrated and isolated. There were times I wanted to get drunk and maudlin, and talk and cry for hours. But I needed someone to do it with, and so couldn't. He expected me to get better far more quickly than I did, and became impatient with having to fetch and carry for me, and taking over while I crawled into my bed with monotonous regularity. It wasn't that he didn't care: he was just optimistic, had never been ill or in hospital, couldn't be objective, and doesn't talk about feelings. This left a gulf between us which has healed. It was a shock, though, to discover that my cancer didn't 'bring us closer'.

The other thing that has come out of my experience is that I have become aware of my potentially high risk of breast cancer. When trying to decide whether or not to keep my ovaries, I was told that if I lost them I'd have to take HRT. This looked bad on two counts: one, all four of my father's sisters have had breast cancer; two, my mother has just been diagnosed with osteoporosis. Exploring the issues around breast cancer led me to a geneticist who worked out my risks and helped me to decide to keep my ovaries. This was hard — in my experience, professionals tend to be totally in favour of HRT, or totally against it — no middle ground. The decision had to be my own. One doctor I spoke to said if I took HRT, I'd "have breast cancer within five years". I didn't particularly believe him, but his strong feelings must have come from somewhere. I'm still going down the genetics route and am potentially considering a prophylactic mastectomy as a preventative measure. Having cancer is 'easy' — both you and your surgeon want to get it out, fast. Trying to cheat a possible future cancer with radical surgery is a difficult and personal gamble, and no-one will make the decision for you because it's too important. Most hereditary breast cancers are also linked to ovarian cancer, so the list goes on for me. All I can say to people is to seek out and make use of as much information and screening as possible.

I have, almost subconsciously, adjusted my perception of the world, life and other people in many ways. Just this week we are getting to know our new adopted son — a six-year old brother for my daughter. That too has been a radical and enriching process — one that people around us call 'brave' (?!), or which they condemn as injurious to our family and our daughter's happiness (assuming that any child who's been in the care system must be a monster who doesn't deserve a chance in life?). It's easy for people who haven't been through what we've been through, and have been able to produce their 'own', complete family, to completely miss the point.

I'm afraid some of these same people present themselves poorly, as un-objective, selfish, and narrow-minded. I've become less tolerant of others in this way, as a result of what I've been through. But I've thoroughly enjoyed the adoption system over the last year and a half, and feel that what I have lost is a displaced child's gain. In fact we have found a genuinely nice, affectionate, bright little boy who has already built a superb relationship with my daughter. My surgeon shows an ongoing interest in our adoption progress, and I've passed information to other patients of his who were, tragically, childless before their hysterectomies. I would heartily recommend exploring adoption to anyone in those circumstances.

Otherwise.... I spend minimal time doing housework, because it's not important. I enjoy my daughter. I gave up my career and, although I'd like to work again when the children are settled at school, I'm no longer aggressively ambitious. I now have the flexibility to choose what to do — without this, my career would have been a hurtling thing I couldn't get off. I don't care what I do as long as it's close to home, stress-free, and fits in with family life. In fact, I now waitress part-time in the evenings, but have lost a (previously very good) friend who felt I was beneath her because of that work. People can be stupid — like the other 'friend' who, after I'd told her I'd been sick due to a stomach bug, joked, "You aren't pregnant, are you?" — just 18 months after my hysterectomy. She'd even been to see me in hospital; it isn't that a funny joke when you've had your fertility ripped out of you, and she's pregnant when she says it. You really find out who your friends are, after cancer, and I'm glad of that. Out with the chaff. Perhaps I should be more tolerant, but there isn't time. Anyway, I've made much better, deeper relationships afterwards.

"For the sake of the children" - Pauline's story

"You've had what operation?!" is the question I am often asked. Not knowing how to continue the conversation without further medical jargon, all I can do is explain in my own way what has happened to me. One fact is certain, if I had not had this strange-sounding surgery (Pelvic Exenteration, P.E.), I would not be here today.

My life changed in 1984, when I was 38. During a visit to a consultant for a minor problem (or so I thought), I started to bleed heavily during the examination. My senses seemed to tell me that the answer to my whispered question "Is it cancer?" would be "Yes, I am afraid it is."

The hospital wanted me to stay with them until major surgery the next week, but I wanted to go home to prepare myself physically and mentally, and be with my family — husband and six children. In some ways this was not such a good idea, as it was so difficult to deal with other people's feelings. I immediately started getting the "does she take sugar?" treatment from people who did not know how to react. One of the things that cheered me up most was a card from friends calling me a "miserable old sod" and promising to treat me as me.

A week later I awoke from an operation to be told that the planned hysterectomy could not be carried out because of the discovery of a sinister-looking tumour lying behind the womb, too large to remove. "That's it," I remember saying, "What do I do now?"

What I hadn't bargained for was the determination of my doctors who assured me there were other options. "Oh no, not radiation." My heart sank when I realised that this was the option they considered best for me. All the myths and old wives tales came flooding into my mind. How on earth would I cope? This was too much.

Heather, my four-year-old, looked straight at me. "Yes, I know you are going into hospital again, Mummy, but don't be frightened. They always make people better." This statement, this trust, this blind faith, made my blood run cold and I cried and sobbed until I thought my heart would break. Suddenly the emotion changed to terrible anger. No way would I allow this disease to rob me of years with the most precious things in my life — my husband, my children. From today the fight was on.

Radiotherapy turned out to be less of an ordeal than I had expected. Of course I had the days when I felt tired and ill and the days when I felt, or was, sick. But, much to the surprise of my friends and neighbours, other days were spent digging the garden, or going on family outings. I started to relax and tried to believe the worst was over. But my cancer was virulent and had not responded fully to the treatment.

Once again I was facing the surgeon who had given the first diagnosis. The tumour had spread to the bowel and possibly the bladder. Stunned, I held onto the chair as he carried on talking, "Our only course of action is to remove everything in the way of the tumour. We will need at least four teams of surgeons to plan and carry out this complicated task." My response was immediate. "Go ahead." I said.

Positive thinking kept me calm. What did it matter if organs had to go? I would still have my eyes, heart and arms to see, love and hug the ones I loved. I was offered counselling, but attended only once. I was asked if I felt "Why me?", when I replied: "No, in fact, why should it be someone else?", I was told that I did not fit the stereotype of someone told they had cancer.

Four months before my fortieth birthday I underwent surgery lasting nine hours. Thanks to the skills and dedication of the surgical team and the support and help of everyone at the hospital, life for me really did begin at forty. Gone was my womb, bladder, bowel, appendix, vagina and rectum, but also gone was the tumour. The surgeon had not warned me that my vagina would be taken — the first I knew of it was when a nurse arrived a week after the operation "to remove the stitches where your vagina used to be". My consultant apparently thought it would be "too much to cope with on top of everything else". He has since changed his mind after I told him to stop under-estimating women. Women can and do cope with all sorts of things in order to be around for their partner and family.

Getting used to a different way of going to the toilet, putting on and changing the small plastic bags was strange at first. The medical equipment looked like an airfix kit with no instructions — which bits went where? But ever-ready advice from nurses trained in this field (stoma nurses) soon enabled it to become just part of my normal daily routine. Meeting people with a colostomy (bowel removal) and people with a urostomy (bladder removal) gave me a great deal of confidence, but I felt different. They had one bag, I had two. The whole question of my altered body image and my sexuality and femininity also had to be addressed and discussed. I desperately needed to talk to someone just like me.

As a result of a letter published in the Colostomy Welfare Group magazine, *Spectrum*, I received letters from all over the country — women who thought they were the only ones in the world like this. We phone and write to each other. We laugh more than we moan as we share our trials and ultimate triumphs. I learnt to drive at forty, anything is possible now! My message to women would be: never be too scared (or busy) to have a smear test, it could save a lot of pain and heartache, and save your life.

Pauline's story has previously been published in BACUP News. Many thanks to the editor for permission to use parts of that article here.

Diary of a silent but deadly disease — Pauline's story (2)

18th July 1994.

It was a beautiful summer day and I was busily creosoting the back garden fence when I realised it was time to get ready to go for my routine smear check. I was tempted not to go, but I knew it was the wrong attitude because I've always been very aware of how lucky we are in this country to have such an excellent screening programme. Also, as a nurse, I knew that any cancer caught in time was treatable, so I decided to be sensible and go for the check up.

After taking the smear the practice nurse checked my cervix and I noticed the look of concern on her face. She told me there was a hardened area on the side of my cervix that she needed the doctor to check. The five minutes I waited for him to come into the room seemed like five hours and in that time my imagination worked over time. He explained that the lump on the side of my cervix needed further investigation and he would arrange a colposcopy.

That evening I told my husband Kev and made out it was nothing to worry about. That night I went to work on the children's ward at the City General hospital as usual. I'd decided to try to carry on as normal for as long as I could, all the time I was aware of just how fragile the apparent normality of my life really was.

I had been a nurse for 18 years and was very aware of the implications of all that had happened that July afternoon. I was fit, well, and tanned after a recent holiday in Spain. It just wasn't possible that I could be ill. I hadn't any symptoms and had never had any gynae problems. All the time I kept trying to convince myself there was nothing wrong and the colposcopy would be the end of this whole unreal episode. All the time these thoughts were racing around in my head I knew that this type of cancer could be silent yet deadly. For the sake of my own sanity and for the sake of my children, husband, family and friends, I decided to push that thought right to the back of my mind and not to allow it to surface again.

4th August 1994.

The results from my smear had come back clear, so when I went along for the colposcopy I was quite confident there would be nothing wrong.

A nurse explained the procedure to me but I couldn't take in what she was saying, I think she realised that and was really kind and patient. Then a doctor went over the details again and told me he would examine my cervix with a microscope, inject a solution and if that was taken up he would then do a biopsy. I was sure it wouldn't get to that stage, I had convinced myself the lump was simply scar tissue resulting from all the stitches I'd had when the children were born.

So when he did in fact need to do a biopsy I got myself into a real state. The procedure was more painful than I'd expected and I nearly fainted, the kindness and support of the nursing staff is something I will never forget and it was at that stage that I cried for first time since it had all began.

When I went to get changed I was shaking like a leaf, the nurse sat and talked and listened to me so that by the time I went back out to Kev, I was quite calm and managed not to worry him. As I left, the doctor said he would get the results within a week. He said I was a most unlikely candidate for any form of cervical cancer. I thanked him and left there wondering how I would get through the long week ahead.

12th August 1994.

The consultant's secretary had telephoned and made an appointment for 12th August. Again, I worked the night before. Kev was already there waiting for me and we sat quietly, both with our own thoughts as we waited for half an hour to be called into the consulting room. When the nurse called my name I jumped and realised how nervous I was, despite trying to convince myself and everyone else that I wasn't worried and was sure everything would be clear.

We were warmly welcomed by the consultant, Mr Smith [Ed. pseudonym] his first words to me, which still stick in my mind were, "Well dear, you haven't got cancer, but I'm afraid you are going to need a hysterectomy."

My mind was in turmoil and I felt confused. I didn't understand what he meant, surely if I hadn't got cancer I would not need such drastic surgery? He quickly went on to explain that due to the results I would go into hospital the following week for a cone biopsy, which basically meant having a deep biopsy. He told me to prepare myself for a hysterectomy in about a month's time. He then asked if we wanted any more children, I said yes, at the same time Kev said no, we laughed. I thought Mr. Smith would say, "Go away and think about it", but instead to my dismay he told us the decision had been made for us. I was aware of not having a say in the matter and I was beginning to feel out of control and frightened.

Before we left the room the consultant showed us the biopsy report which I read but couldn't take in properly, although I did remember reading the words 'adenocarcinoma in situ' and made a mental note to look it up when I got home.

All along I'd fought back the tears and although shell shocked, Kev was trying to be strong for me. Back at the car I told him I wasn't going to have a hysterectomy and no one could make me, I hadn't got cancer so it wasn't justified. We were both baffled by the consultant's words, telling me I hadn't got cancer yet he was insisting I had major surgery, it didn't add up. Back home I looked in my nursing dictionary and the definition of adenocarcinoma in situ is:— 'A malignant new growth of glandular epithelial tissue in its original position.'

18th August 1994.

Last night I'd taken Katie to her friend's house where she was staying for two days. She cried when I left her. I'd tried to keep life as normal as possible over the past few weeks, but she was an intelligent eleven-year old who, although I had explained things briefly and simply, knew something wasn't quite right. On the way to hospital Kev and I dropped William off at my Mum's, thankfully at six and a half years old he was quite oblivious to any disruption in our lives and was enjoying the fuss Nana made of him!

At 9 a.m. I booked into the ward. The consultant came to see me, explained the procedure involved with a cone biopsy, which seemed quite straightforward, and asked me to sign the consent form.

At 11.30 a.m. a hospital porter quickly took me through the long, brightly lit corridors to the operating theatre. I was unaware of being taken back to the ward but I remember waking up there in severe pain. The consultant was standing over me saying something about "having to remove your whole cervix", "a bigger operation than expected", "you will definitely need a hysterectomy", "another appointment next week". I responded with "I can't stand this pain, please give me something". He was quite concerned and went to find a nurse.

I was given distalgesics but they did nothing, she offered more morphine but I refused it, I hated how it made me feel. So she gave Volterol suppositories and eventually the pain subsided. Kev came to see me, I was really pleased to see him and tried to tell him what the consultant had said but the painless sleep I'd craved drifted over me like a big soft blanket and I willingly snuggled into it.

By the time I woke up late that afternoon, I felt a lot better, the pain was much easier but I felt groggy from the anaesthetic. I was really thirsty and drank glass after glass of water. I also managed some soup and a yoghurt. The other ladies in the ward were chatty and that helped pass the time. I began to feel very sorry for myself as one by one they were discharged home, they'd had D & Cs or been sterilised and I was the only one who had had an operation for cancer.

Mr Smith called back to see me and was glad the pain had settled, again he told me I'd have to have a hysterectomy in a month's time, I think he realised I wasn't accepting this and so he kept telling me. He explained that by removing my cervix he was sure he had cleared the cancer cells. "Surely then I won't need a hysterectomy." I said. "It all depends on the histology report, which I will have when I see you in outpatients next week." he explained gently. "But," he went on, "Whatever the report says, under the circumstances, if it were my wife, I would want her to have the surgery." With that he squeezed my hand, smiled kindly and went.

My colleagues from the children's ward all took turns to come up and see me. Most of them were shocked to find I'd had an operation and was due for major surgery within a month. A week or two earlier I had been working with them and seemed perfectly fit and healthy. I'd never been off sick from work before and wasn't even sure how to fill out a sick note.

Before leaving the ward I'd been given an appointment to see the consultant again in a week's time. Over the next seven days I took Brufen and distalgesics for constant pain. I felt floaty and too weak to do normal household chores. Friends and family visited and phoned every day while neighbours picked the children up from school. I began to believe there was something seriously wrong, why else would I be feeling so ill and be in so much pain?

26th August 1994.

Again Kev and I went to outpatients together. We waited over half an hour and I was in a lot of pain. Eventually we were called into the consultant's room, but were disappointed to be told the histology results hadn't come back. Mr Smith examined me to see why I was in so much pain and told me I'd got an infection. He wrote a prescription for antibiotics and told us to go and have a cup of tea while he rang for the results. Over a drink I confided in Kev that I was sure there was something very wrong, he just squeezed my hand. There was nothing he could say, I know he feared the worst too. We had been married for seventeen years and he had never seen me ill before.

When we were next called in to Mr Smith's room, he told us: "I'm afraid the cancer cells are more invasive than first thought. They have been found on the outside edges of the biopsy, which was basically your whole cervix, we can't be sure how much further they have advanced." He paused, to give us chance to absorb what he was saying. Kev and I sat silently looking at him and waiting to hear what else he had to say. "I'm going to refer you to a colleague of mine, Mr Jones a gynae-oncologist who specialises in your condition. He will perform an operation called a Wertheim's hysterectomy, which involves removal of your womb, ovaries, abdominal lymph glands, perimetrium and part of the vagina." He talked slowly and clearly, making allowance for our sense of shock. The tears pricked at the side of my eyes and I asked why this had happened to me, what had I done to cause it? He insisted none of it was my fault and I was just very, very unlucky. I looked at Kev and saw the tears in his eyes. I didn't want to break down, I wanted to try and remember everything that was being said. I needed to think it through and get it all straight in my mind before the onslaught of inevitable questions from all my family and friends who were waiting for me to let them know how this appointment had gone.

Kev had to go back to work. I drove back to my in-law's house but the children had gone out with their aunt. I was really upset and dreaded going back to my own empty house. As I let myself in the through the front door the cold silence engulfed me and I felt very, very sorry for myself.

As I expected the phone was soon ringing, a work friend, I told her what had been said, then my sister Kath rang and I told her, for the first time I sobbed and she cried too. "It's just not fair." she kept saying.

Kath had been invited to Wales for the weekend, but she rang me to say she wasn't going and would be coming over to spend the evening with me. I knew she was looking forward to seeing her friends in Wales. Kath had lived there before her husband's untimely death from cancer at the age of 46, leaving her a widow with two children at only 36 years old. She insisted that she wouldn't enjoy it and didn't feel up to the journey, I had to admit I would be glad of her company.

Kev fetched fish and chips for tea and I managed to eat a little bit. By then I was feeling exhausted and had become concerned about the amount of blood I had been losing since Mr Smith had examined me. I didn't say anything to any one but decided that if it didn't stop soon I would give the ward a ring for some advice.

William was happily playing with his box of Lego and Kev was busy decorating the bedroom. About 7 p.m. my Mum phoned from my other sister's home in Wiltshire. I made light of how I felt and told her I'd know more about my operation the following week. There was no point in worrying her and there was nothing she could do anyway. I placed the receiver down and just then I felt a sudden surge of warm fluid on my legs, looking down I saw blood seeping through my jeans. In a blind panic I jumped of the settee, ran upstairs and shouted to Kev to phone for an ambulance. When he saw me he went white and nearly passed out, the children came running out of their bedroom and I suddenly felt guilty for frightening them. Kev had rung for an ambulance and I told him to ring his Mum and ask her to come up. His hands were shaking so much he could hardly press the buttons. Then I told him to phone Kath and ask her to meet us at the accident unit.

It seemed an age before the ambulance arrived. At the same time that it pulled into the drive Kev's brother Michael arrived with his Mum. I felt better when I knew the children had someone to look after them. The ambulance men carried me down stairs and I heard William try to comfort Katie who was crying. He told her not to worry as Mummy would be all right, "She's only having a baby." I could still cry now when I think about the irony of what he'd said. He was six and a half years old.

Once in the ambulance I was given oxygen and was attached to a machine that monitored my oxygen levels. We made the same journey I had made earlier that day but this time I had left my children upset and bewildered and I was travelling with Kev in an ambulance driving at top speed with the sirens going. It all felt very unreal, like a bad dream that I would wake up from any minute.

I was put in a cubicle, a nurse came in and checked my blood pressure. Otherwise I just lay there for what seemed like hours. An excruciating pain had built up in my abdomen and when I could stand it no more Kev went and looked for a nurse. For hours I had put off going to the toilet because I was afraid of making the bleeding worse, so I thought the pain was a full bladder. The nurse helped me on to the bed pan and I passed a huge clot that felt like giving birth to a full sized baby. Taking the pan away the nurse looked quite shocked. I became upset and wondered how much more blood I could lose before I died! Kath calmed me down. Poor Kev, he hates hospitals and illness. It must have been so awful for him.

Kev has since told me that he thought I was going to die. He said my face and lips were grey. When Mr Jones' registrar arrived he immediately took control of the situation. The theatre was closed for the night so he rang nursing staff and an anaesthetist to come in and open it. He asked me to sign a consent form which gave him permission to perform the Wertheim's hysterectomy if he could not stop the haemorrhaging. I didn't want to sign it, I'd only been told about the Wertheim's that morning and before then I had never heard of it. I needed longer to find out what was involved and accept it. Kev and Kath encouraged me to sign and helped me to hold the pen.

I remember looking at the faces around my bed, the registrar, two nurses, Kath and Kev, all eagerly waiting for me to sign so I could be taken to theatre. I looked at them and thought, "They are all more worried about me dying than I am." I know the Pethidine was partly responsible for my feeling of euphoria, but I was genuinely accepting of my own death. I knew the children would miss me, but they would be well looked after and I had guided them through their babyhood and given them the love and care that would stand them in good stead for the rest of their lives. I had lost my Dad two years earlier and missed him terribly. My faith meant I felt content in the thought my Dad was waiting for me. I wasn't frightened.

The operation went ahead and it seemed like seconds later when I heard my name being called, I opened my eyes and seeing the nurse, said, "Hello Vicky." Everyone laughed and Kev and Kath entered the room to the sound of laughter which was a great relief to them. I was relieved to know I hadn't had the hysterectomy. The doctor said it was best that I didn't have it done then as I was too weak for such major surgery.

The ward I worked on was downstairs and when they heard I had been admitted one of the nurses, Gill, came up and sat with me. It was strange having her there moistening my lips and caring for me, when only two weeks earlier we had been working together. I slept until morning and woke up feeling groggy. I don't remember much about that day except that Mr Jones came to see me. He explained all about the Wertheim's hysterectomy to me and why it was essential. He said I wouldn't be strong enough for it for at least another month. I needed to get over the two anaesthetics I'd had in quick succession and build up my iron levels after the haemorrhage.

I recovered well and when my Mum came with my sister June on the Sunday evening they were both surprised and pleased to see how well I was looking. The nursing staff said they were confident I would make a good and quick recovery when I eventually had the hysterectomy.

31st August 1994.

I'd bled again in the night and when Mr Jones came to see me he arranged for blood to be cross-matched ready and sent me for x-rays in case I needed the Wertheim's as an emergency. He said it was the last thing he wanted to do but he might not have a choice! I was really, really upset. I rang Kath and asked her to take a day off work. After coming to the ward to see me she went to my house to help Kev with the cleaning, washing and shopping.

Mr Smith called to see me and hadn't realised all that had gone on and was upset to see me so low, I was really weepy that day. One of the other patients had helped me a lot and I'd come to depend on her emotionally. When she went home that afternoon I broke my heart.

That night like the next few days were uneventful so by Saturday I was well enough to go home. It was lovely to feel so much better but as I said goodbye to the other patients and thanked all the nurses I had the awful thought of knowing I had to go back in on 4th October for the Wertheim's.

The month passed quickly but I enjoyed doing the things I hadn't had the time to do when I was working. I caught up with friends and hardly a day went by when someone didn't come for lunch. I built myself up, put back the one and half stone I'd lost since all this began and by the time October came I was feeling well and relaxed. We made arrangements for Katie and William to be cared for after school while I was in hospital. Other than that we hadn't talked a lot about it. We'd managed to keep the normality in our lives that I'd hoped for. Then on the morning of 3rd October I dropped them off at school, they gave me a kiss and skipped into the playground like it was any ordinary day. I felt really proud of them and was relieved there had been no tears.

4th October 1994.

I woke up after a good night's sleep feeling surprisingly calm. The time of the operation was brought forward from 1pm to 11.30am. I quickly rang Kev, had a bath, put on a theatre gown and took my premeds. Soon after I became drowsy and pleasantly relaxed. My Mum and Kath came and sat with me until a porter came and wheeled me down to the theatre. The months of waiting were over and now I just wanted to get through the operation and go back home to my family. It wasn't with fear that I was taken into theatre, it was with relief.

Later that afternoon I woke up in the HDU (High Dependency Unit). Kev was with me and said I'd been awake on and off for an hour. He'd been to a seminar in the morning and I kept asking him how it had gone! As well as feeling drunk I was shivering uncontrollably and was wrapped in a space blanket. I had tubes everywhere and was attached to several monitors. Kev went to pick the children up from his Mum's and we agreed he wouldn't bring them to see me until the next day.

I slept on and off throughout the night and every time I woke a nurse was sitting with me and constantly monitoring my condition. By morning I had an unbearable headache. Later it was explained to me that when the epidural had been injected into my spine, cerebral fluid had leaked out. I was told that the horrendous headache I was experiencing would stay with me for at least five days. I felt I couldn't stand it, for five more minutes never mind five days, it was as though my skull was being slowly pulled apart.

The staff were very caring and did everything they could to reduce the pain. I had regular analgesics and a cold compress on my forehead. One of the nurses lent me his sunglasses because I couldn't stand the light. Every sound I heard was amplified, so even though the HDU was generally quiet I couldn't stand all the noises around me. It was decided that the best thing to do was to transfer me back to a side room on the ward where it would be easier to keep me in quiet darkness. I was kept pain free with Pethidine and was given regular anti-sickness injections. Another symptom of the leaked spinal fluid was constant nausea and vomiting on the slightest movement. I just took sips of water and was on a drip to replace my sugars and salts.

Kev brought the children to see me for the first time since before the operation and William didn't want to come in the room. It upset me but I could understand how hard it must be for a six year old to comprehend. I had to lie flat and keep my eyes shut, there were still lots of tubes attached, it must have been very frightening for him. Katie accepted it better and she brought me a lovely drawing that she had done of Winnie the Pooh and the nurses put it up on the wall.

I had a drug-induced good night's sleep but hated waking up to the constant headache and awful sickly feeling. After a bed bath and a change of nightie I felt a lot better. The drain was taken out of my wound which initially was a relief, but soon after I was very sick and had to be cleaned up again. When the nurses had done all that I looked in the bed and saw I was swimming in blood which had leaked from the drain site. I was so upset, all the bed had to be stripped and I was washed and changed once again. Soon after, my mother and sister-in-law visited, I was exhausted and weak. Kev hadn't told them about the problems the epidural had caused so they expected me to be sitting up and able to chat to them.

8th October 1994.

Tubes were going one by one, my headache was slightly better and I could tolerate a dim light. Mr Jones came in, sat on my bed and told me how well the operation had gone. He explained that it had only taken two hours instead of the expected three. He said everything looked clear although he couldn't be totally sure until the histology came back, which would take about five days.

I made slow but sure progress over the next two days, but the nights were long and despite having sleeping tablets I hardly slept. Each day I did a little bit more. I had a bath, sat out for an hour or two, wrote a few letters and had more tubes removed. A nurse gently took the metal clips out of my wound, which thankfully was healing well. The anaesthetist who had given me the epidural, came to see me and as he went out of the door, he turned back and said sorry.

Seven days after the operation I was feeling really low and wondering when I'd ever begin to feel well again. That day I was very, very sick, when the nurse came in she just stood open mouthed. It took them ages to clean up and even the curtains had to be changed!!

I felt rotten for the rest of the day, but had a good nights sleep and when I woke next morning, lo and behold, MY HEADACHE HAD GONE. I couldn't believe it, I kept expecting it to come back but it didn't. My headache went and my appetite came back with a vengeance. The nurses were thrilled and brought me extra helpings. I rang Kev and told him the good news. As soon as I saw the Sister I told her I felt well enough to go home.

13th October 1994.

I was told my histology results were all clear and I wouldn't need any further treatment except a regular check up at outpatients. Mr Jones had told me he was sure everything would be okay, but now I had it in writing and allowed myself to believe it. I was aware of how very lucky I was not to need a course of radiotherapy or chemotherapy, although two years earlier I would have been given radiotherapy as a precautionary measure, now research showed that it hadn't proved to be of any benefit.

I was home by late afternoon. My Mum welcomed me and the house looked lovely. Kev had almost finished papering the sitting room, Mum had tidied all through, and the dinner was cooking in the oven. Kev went to his Mum's and fetched Katie and William home. Katie ran to me and we had a lovely cuddle. William was a bit distant but as the evening went on he snuggled up to me and was his usual loving self.

That night it was wonderful to sleep in my own bed. I appreciated all the things I had always taken for granted and was seeing everything through different eyes. I drifted to sleep thanking God for my health, my home, my lovely family and many friends.

February 1998.

It's now three and a half years since my operation and I'm perfectly well and enjoying a busy, active life. Katie and William are growing up fast and I often look at them and think how lucky I am to see them grow up. I know that if the practice nurse hadn't found that lump when she did it would all be a very different story.

I went back to Mr Jones at outpatients for three years before being discharged under the care of my GP. I know if I have any problems or worries I can ring Mr Jones' secretary and she'll make an appointment for me to see him. I have HRT patches and find they suit me better than taking a tablet every day.

I left the children's ward soon after returning to work and became a Marie Curie nurse. I never tell patients that I've had cancer but my experience helps me to understand the fears they and their families have. I've recently started working as a district nurse and am starting an 18 month course in April. I'm enjoying my work and am looking

forward to the course and all the opportunities the
qualification of RGN will bring.

In May last year I was 40 years old and threw a party
as a way of thanking my family and friends for all the support
Kev and I were given when I was ill. I told everyone I didn't
want presents but they could give a donation to the Douglas
Macmillan Hospice where my Dad had been cared for four
and a half years earlier. A conservatory is being built at the
hospice this year and I am providing a fountain with the
money from my party. I explained to all my friends and
family that I didn't want presents because I've got everything
I want. I have my health, two beautiful children, a good
husband and a lovely home. All the things money can't buy
and all the things I now appreciate and enjoy so much.

I know full well that if I hadn't gone along for that check
smear back in July 1994 the cancerous lump found by the
nurse would have spread to my ovaries and become a fatal
illness. I will be forever grateful to her and to all the medical
profession who worked so hard to successfully cure me of
the silent yet deadly disease of cervical cancer.

Rosemary's story

I suppose I knew in the back of my mind: I had been a
nurse and I now work as a practice manager for the local
GPs. I had been on the contraceptive pill for years and
convinced myself that the change in my menstrual cycle was
due to being pre-menopausal. By May 1996 I started to
experience post coital bleeding, abdominal and low back
pain and my periods went haywire. In July I realised I was
relying on Paracetamol every day but I really wanted to get
through August — I was judging at a canine championship

show at Bournemouth then (our hobby - breeding, exhibiting and judging pugs). My back ached, I had a dragging sensation in my lower abdomen, I had cramp in my thighs, was bleeding heavily virtually all the time and my bottom felt numb!

By September I felt I had to give in and approached my female GP who is also my employer. She was kindness itself. I had a smear taken and sent to Mediscreen privately, a blood test, and on examination she thought the mass in the left adnexa she felt could be a fibroid or ovarian cyst. Perhaps it was the way I looked at her because she added "or something more sinister". She got on the telephone to organise an appointment with a gynaecologist, and I asked to go privately (we had insurance for years and only used it once).

The smear came back showing borderline changes and my haemoglobin was down a bit. I saw the consultant gynaecologist on 1st October 1996. He spoke frankly, and I thanked him for it. He considered that the growth was highly suspicious and he wanted me in for EUA, hysteroscopy, D and C, cervical biopsy and diagnostic cystoscopy on 3rd October. I had heard good reports of him and on meeting him I was happy to trust his opinion. His secretary organised everything for me and asked me to ring her if I had any queries.

I reported to the Private Hospital with my overnight bag at 7.15 a.m. and by 10 a.m. I was on my way to theatre. By the time I had fully come round in the afternoon I was slightly sore but otherwise okay. The consultant came to see me that evening and sat on the bed by my side. It was confirmed — I had stage 2b squamous cell carcinoma of the cervix. A stillness swept over me whilst I absorbed the fact, the doctor held my hand and although he was talking I could not hear his words.

Eventually I picked up on "radiotherapy proved just as good if not better than operation, 40% survival rate at five years on". I then began to ask questions and he slowly talked me through it all again and whilst promising nothing he seemed optimistic. He left and a nurse came in and I just broke down. During that night on my own in that hospital bed I felt emotions like I never have before. I was frightened, angry, depressed. Please remove this alien thing from my body, take it away, I did not invite it here. I left the following day with an appointment for a CT scan on 11th October.

At work on the Monday I told a few colleagues. They had to know, after all I would be off sick, but it was also a relief to tell someone. I am sure some felt that I was wrong to talk about it, some people seemed embarrassed but most were great and very supportive. Thoughts went round inside my head, I felt cold, took my two Co-codamol every six hours, worked my way through the following days on autopilot, concentration came and went again. My husband sorted out his work shifts and also told a few people, his sister, and our daughter. I think he had to offload the news as much as I had to.

Why me? What had I done wrong? My family did not deserve this. Cancer shouted out at me from everywhere — in the newspapers, on television, conversations and at work. Fear sometimes overwhelmed me and I just cried and cried. Guilt consumed me — I should have had smear tests, stopped the pill, given up smoking, had a better diet — I beat myself up at every opportunity. I read all I could get my hands on concerning cancer, some good and some bad. It did not really help. I just felt depressed and confused by some of the technical jargon in the medical books. I had nursed old ladies with this and they were so very ill — some 25 years ago!

The CT scan was an experience. Drink what seems like gallons of sour syrup and don't go to the loo! At least you get to keep your underwear on, you do start to get the urge to take off your clothes every time someone in a white coat approaches! It was fascinating to think that the folk behind the screen were looking at pictures of the inside of me, and I concentrated on the machinery so as not to panic.

A week later I had a chance meeting with our Macmillan nurse at the surgery where I work. I blurted out the news, and we chatted for a while. I shall always remember her words — its sink or swim, just think swim, be strong and fight all the way — and she gave me the address of BACUP. The booklets that I requested were read from cover to cover and I found them so practical and full of advice. I referred to them many times.

On the 30th October 1996 I had my first appointment with the consultant oncologist, with his female registrar in attendance too. He discussed with me and my husband all the findings and the treatment he wanted to offer. John left and I was examined by the consultant who then also left but the female registrar stayed on to talk. She went through things again and we talked at some length about the external beam and intracavity radiotherapy, acute and long term side effects, hormone replacement therapy and the use of vaginal dilators to keep the vagina patent. The consultant appeared again to say the simulator was free if I wanted to get on with things and then the radiotherapy could start the following day. The simulator was an uncomfortable experience. Basically it is the same as the linear accelerator machine that would deliver the radiotherapy but instead takes measurements, marks positions on your body, etc. It meant having a medium rather like a tampon inserted and positioning in weird postures whilst everyone left the room and the lights went out — I just kept thinking "keep your sense of humour!".

The following day started my 20 fractions of external beam radiotherapy. Every day Monday to Friday for 20 days. It roughly took 3 hours travelling time there and back. I had been offered a hostel stay as we lived that far from the hospital but I am pleased I stayed at home with my husband as his support was so very important to my well-being. The treatments were painless and quick. All I had to do was lay face down on a table, the radiographer adjusted my position then left the room, the lights went out and the machine made all the right noises and movements. The beam seemed to be directed at my lower back first and then the machine moved under me to target my pubic region. A radio played low music in the background and within minutes it was over — "see you tomorrow". The radiographers were so nice and always asked about symptoms of side effects.

I saw a doctor once a week but if there was a problem a doctor always seemed to be about in the department. I managed to get to work for about five hours a day during the next four weeks of treatment. During this time I had to have a check chest x-ray and blood test, and got to know a few of the staff and regular patients. Everyone was cheerful and the department was bright and airy. The tiredness began to tell, a combination I think of radiotherapy, travelling and working. By the 17th day I felt exhausted and my skin was red and itchy, and pubic hair was a thing of the past! I had suffered from bouts of diarrhoea and nausea but was given plenty of medication to overcome these problems. On the plus side the bleeding had stopped and the pains had gone. My ovaries had been zapped, as they promised they would. I decided to give work a miss and was taken up to the ward where I was to be admitted on the 20th day, shown around, even the bed I would have and the machines. After the 20th external treatment I went up to that ward, was clerked in, saw the anaesthetist, consultant and all the usual paraphernalia was explained. I sat by my bed wondering if I ran away would anyone notice!

The following day was taken up with preparations for theatre. I was to have three applicators inserted into my vagina with packing holding all in place, along with a catheter to exclude the need to get up to go to the loo — Codeine in large quantities had taken care of the other bodily function! After this it was back to the simulator to check the positioning was good and then in to my bed on the ward.

The physicist, with a doctor, arrived to set up the machine called Selectron — a Dalek type of creature. The tubes from the Selectron are fixed to the applicators, necessary figures are programmed in and switched on and the caesium pellets are passed into the applicators, if the machine is switched off or someone enters the area the pellets are withdrawn back into the machine. The protective barriers go up and I had to lay there for 12 hours. Admittedly I was given Morphine, lovely iced water to drink and plenty of hand waving from the other side of the barrier. Flowers from my boss had awaited my arrival and they cheered me up no end. I listened to an audio book about a train journey which actually kept my mind quite occupied between sleeping and having my back carefully rubbed by the nurses who quickly came and went so as not to prolong their exposure time. I just kept thinking "squirm you rotten cells." Removing the applicators when the time was up took two nurses, a jab of Morphine and gritted teeth.

The following bath was heaven but I felt that I would never cross my legs ever again. The pain was almost intolerable and going to the toilet a nightmare. I saw the Cancer Nurse Specialist who talked so much sense and reality. She explained the use of the dilators and I was to learn later how important these things were to keep my female bits working properly!

The next two weeks left me drained and miserable although this was considered time off. I stayed at home feeling sore in any position and just generally low. As the days passed I found myself probably at my lowest ebb. I cried a lot, slept at all the wrong times, laying awake at night and looked dreadful. I was only comfortable in a warm bath. Was this it then, was I never going to feel any better than this.

On the 11th December I went in for the second internal treatment — but 25 hours this time. I do not know how I controlled my fear. It seems irrational now but then I could have gone berserk. Same procedure but on getting up from the bed I was awfully sick this time due to laying flat for so long. The oncologist told me that the gynaecologist had been present in theatre this time and that they had got the applicators in a better position.

I came home to flowers and cards everywhere. I treasure the words from my friends via letters and telephone calls. I really had to try hard and not let these people down. My husband had been great all the way along. All the sayings spring to mind — tower of strength, shoulder to cry on etc. but I really do not know what I would have done without him, in fact he probably took all my anguish on board and began to look quite ill himself. After 26 years of marriage he knows me so well. I am sure my daughter suffered too although I tried to hide my despair from her.

Fortunately my dogs had to be exercised, this made me walk round our field, even if the weather was cold and the ground frozen for weeks. My dear pugs must have thought I had gone mad as I actually enjoyed watching my breath in the cold air and the foot marks left in the frost.

I began to talk myself round and feeling better I went back to work in January after eight weeks off sick. I read books on visualisation and imagery, diet and other self help techniques. Whilst I have not practised every detail certain things I have picked out have helped me a great deal.

I was on the three monthly follow up regime at outpatients. I have had a couple of hiccoughs — urinary tract infection and itchy skin but with the help of my GP these have been treated. Its strangely nice to have the hospital doctors confirm that all is settling down because I now feel quite well. In fact I sometimes almost forget that I have cancer, its not been removed, the invader is still there as part of me but I do not want it to overtake me and have control. I have often thought of writing it all down and it has been very therapeutic and cleansing.

I have just been for a hospital check up and saw the oncologist and a gynae-registrar. Both examined me and independently agreed that the big mass that was recorded on my first examination, before treatment, was no longer palpable and all that could be felt was scar tissue from the radiotherapy. I go back in 4 months time.

I feel very well and psychologically much better. My whole perspective on life has changed. Certain things mean nothing now and others things mean everything. Why do we whine and moan about trivia, we are wasting time and should get on with living. I am packing into my life all the things I want to do. I am happy and alive.

Sue's story

I was told that I had cervical cancer on the Saturday before Christmas 1994. I initially went to see my doctor because I was bleeding after intercourse. My doctor did a smear test and also referred me for a hospital appointment. At the colposcopy clinic the consultant took a sample and advised me that he was not particularly happy with what he found and would contact me following the biopsy.

I received a telephone call on the Friday night at home asking me to go into hospital at 4 p.m. on the Saturday as the consultant wanted to see me. The nurse on the phone wouldn't or couldn't give any further information so it was very scary — we knew something was obviously wrong. I went in with my husband and the consultant broke the news — he saw us in a private room. He was initially very apologetic, he explained everything and gave us his home number in case we wanted to talk over the weekend. I was left with no doubt that surgery was the only option. He referred me to a second consultant as he himself could not do the operation.

I saw the second consultant on the Wednesday and talked everything through with him. He drew diagrams and gave me as much time as I wanted. He arranged for me to see 'Mary' a previous patient, as he thought I would find it useful. Before admission to hospital I also had a lengthy talk with my GP. 'Mary' came to see me in hospital the day before my operation. She bounded into the ward — happy, healthy, and full of life — and showed me that there was life after this. Her example became my 'goal' to achieve.

The operation was a success, though the ten days in hospital were a nightmare — I dislike hospitals having had two previous lengthy stays (not cancer-related). However my mother had contacted everyone who knew me and I ended up with about eighty cards, enough flowers to fill the ward, daily pictures from my son Adam, balloons on the bed rail, etc., etc. The nurses remarked that all I needed was some flashing lights and it would look like the Blackpool illuminations!

The family had planned a surprise party for when I arrived home — and this was all Adam would talk about when he came to visit. I got the news that the lymph glands were clear on the day I was discharged, my family were ecstatic, but I felt numb. I had at first been quite strong, I didn't really cry, I was rather matter-of-fact about the whole thing, "what do we do now?" attitude, "let's get on and sort it out". This continued for about the first couple of weeks at home. We had our party and then my sister and her daughter came to stay to help me out, and as company for Adam. But after a few weeks depression hit — and did it hit!!

I was well-supported by work friends, family and my own doctor, and although I wasn't under any pressure to return to work I was desperate to do so in order to prove to myself that I was all right again. However, an understanding husband who was prepared to make hot chocolate and talk at three in the morning, and a course of Prozac, helped the most. The depression did not lift easily, I would say that it has taken a good twelve months or longer for me to mentally accept that I have had cancer — I found that, and thoughts of death the hardest things to cope with. But hopefully all is well now — and I can now smile and sing and enjoy life again.

My ideas to help:

1. Before an operation (or other treatment) — is there anyone you can see who has been through it themselves? — ask your consultant.

2. Make sure everyone knows you are going into hospital — the more cards the merrier, they make you feel good and that you are not forgotten.

3. Plan a welcome home party — something to talk about and look forward to.

4. Don't be too hard on yourself and don't expect too much from yourself. Set achievable targets, be it work or home or relationships.

5. Talk to your doctors and consultants, make sure you know what they are talking about. You have a right to as much or as little information as you want. You are a person, not just a file.

6. Come to terms with death, it will happen to us all sooner or later. You are not the only one.

7. It does get easier. Expect good days and bad days. But isn't it wonderful when the sun shines!

Tess's story

I was diagnosed with cervical cancer in January 1997 at the age of 51. I had started to have a clear, watery discharge in November 1996, and hoped that 'it would go away', however by early January the discharge had turned a pinkish colour, which was when I first when to my GP. She thought it was just a post-menopausal symptom (I had an early menopause at 44), particularly as my last smear test four years previously had been clear, as had all the others preceding it. However she referred me to a gynaecologist at the local NHS hospital. Despite my GP's optimism, I 'knew' it was cancer and, after two weeks without receiving an appointment from the hospital, I phoned and said I wanted to be seen privately, and was, two days later.

The lady gynaecologist at the private hospital was very kind and began by saying that she had no intention of hurting me. The examination by my GP had been very uncomfortable so this piece of news was much welcome! She said: "Ah, yes, the bleeding's coming from....the cervix....oh!" The instrument she was using got caught on the tumour and a lump of it came away. She was very keen to show me this lump in its specimen jar and said; "It doesn't look very good, does it?" I asked if it could be anything other than cancer, and she repeated "It doesn't look very good."

I had to wait another week for the pathology results and, unfortunately, by that time had convinced myself that I didn't have cancer — so when I walked in it was a shock when she said "It's what you and I knew it was." I felt like shouting "NO!"

Following the diagnosis I was seen within a few days at the Royal Marsden, Fulham, as an NHS patient. I was then taken in the following week for an examination under general anaesthetic, at which time it was decided to treat me surgically, rather than with radiotherapy. The following week I had a radical hysterectomy, as well as the removal of two sets of lymph nodes. An epidural was put in place for any pain but I asked for this to be removed the third day, post op, because I felt so awful. Apart from quite bad 'wind' pains I was fortunate in not having any pain that I can remember. However, on the seventh day after the operation, I began to lose a lot of clear fluid, which quite literally poured away. No one really seemed sure exactly what it was but the surgeon thought it may be lymph. Apparently this was quite an unusual thing to happen. The next day it stopped but started again the following day, but this time a colour like Tizer!

I went home a fortnight after the operation, which may have been a little longer than some other ladies, but possibly because I had a temperature (104) most days. When I left hospital I was told that, as far as they could tell, I would not need any further treatment as both ovaries and the lymph nodes were clear of cancer. So it came as quite a shock when, at my first outpatient check-up five weeks later, I was told I needed radiotherapy because they had found pre-cancerous cells at the top of the vagina. At first, I was told that it would be four doses of internal radiotherapy.

At that stage I telephoned the Bristol Cancer Help Centre and spoke to a lady doctor who said it wouldn't hurt if I put off the radiotherapy for three months and tried some complementary treatment. This consisted of mega-vitamins, and douching myself every day with a herb called golden rod. I was unsure of whether to follow this advice or not, but two days later my mind was made up for me. The Marsden told me that, as well as the pre-cancerous cells, pathology had shown cancer cells within the pelvic area. This meant that I would need five weeks of external radiotherapy, on a daily basis, followed by two internal appointments.

I certainly don't regret my decision to go ahead with the radiotherapy immediately. The radiotherapists were really lovely people, I was always seen on time, and was offered plenty of help with any problems which the radiotherapy might cause. I felt slightly nauseous the first couple of days but that passed. I had loose bowels from about the second week. I was very apprehensive about the internal radiotherapy, but in the event, there were no problems at all, soft music in the background, no pain or even discomfort — if only going to the dentist were that pleasant! I was fortunate in that I did not have any burning of the skin around the pelvic area; I did lose my pubic hair but this has since grown back.

However, I do now have a problem with oedema (fluid) in the pubic area and lower stomach. I was originally told at an outpatient appointment that this was because I'm fair-skinned, blue-eyed, and had lost two sets of lymph nodes. I was also told to massage the area. I tried this but it didn't make any appreciable difference. For some weeks in the summer of '97 I went to an acupuncturist, primarily for help with the oedema, but have since found out that this is not to be recommended. However, the acupuncturist suggested putting tiny magnets on the scar and this did seem to promote healing of the external scar tissue. Some months after the pelvic oedema first appeared, my left leg, ankle and foot swelled up. At first I didn't associate this with the oedema but that was what it was. I was going to a reflexologist and told her about it; after two sessions of reflexology the swelling in my left leg went completely and has not returned, however the reflexology has not made any difference to the pelvic lymphoedema.

Since then I have been in contact with the Lymphoedema Clinic at the Royal Marsden, and had an appointment in December '97, which was very useful in terms of self-care of the affected area. At the time of writing (March '98) I am about to start a week's treatment of manual lymphatic drainage, as a private patient, and have just bought a pair of £18 Marks & Spencers' pants to give strong support to the relevant area (similar ones in another chain store were £30!). The nurse who is to do the MLD (manual lymphatic drainage) has suggested I take up swimming again, as this is an excellent exercise for this particular problem. I also go regularly to a therapeutic healer: if nothing else, this seems to help keep my spirits up.

I have to use a vaginal dilator (supplied by the hospital), as I do not have a sexual partner. Apparently the combination of being post-menopausal and having radiotherapy, means that the vagina closes up so, sex apart, internal examinations would otherwise become very difficult.

I have read that cancer of the cervix is caused by a virus, similar to some venereal diseases. I was with my late husband (who died of prostate cancer) for nearly 15 years, no one else, and I find the idea upsetting and distasteful, but have to own up to a few wild years, so unfortunately the multi-partner theory may well be true. Perhaps this knowledge could be stressed to today's young people!

So, just over a year on from the operation, how do I feel? Physically, strong and well, but mentally and emotionally, not so good. I realise that I no longer buy any attractive clothes, just functional things, and although I have put on a stone in weight this last year, and am now heavier than at any time before, I do not seem to have the interest to do anything about it. Although I was sterilised when 25, it was only after this hysterectomy 26 years later that I feel less of a woman, sometimes when I am walking in the street now, I seem to be almost invisible! As regards fearing that the cancer may return, there are times when I am very, very afraid, but fortunately they are not too common. Some months ago I went to a Cancerlink group and although they were friendly and welcoming, I realised that sitting in a circle talking about myself was not for me. However, my brother who lives in France has cancer, and occasionally I have spoken to him about how I feel, particularly about these feelings of blind panic, and he seems to understand completely. It does help to be able to talk to someone who doesn't feel 'embarrassed' because they are not in the same boat!

Afterword - Mikki and Brian's Story

Mikki first wrote to me in October 1996. She had just been diagnosed with cervical cancer and had contacted BACUP for advice. As well as booklets, they had sent her the newsletter with my request for contacts for this book, and she had responded straight away.

Her cancer was found after she insisted on investigation following a clear smear test. She had been suffering back pain and it was thought it might have been a kidney stone. She wrote:

"On 4th October I had the ultrasound. My kidneys and ovaries appeared normal but there was something else on the scan. The doctor was called by the operator and he looked as well. He asked when I had my last smear (14th July) and since that had been clear suggested that this was a fibroid. I saw my GP later that day and asked whether my smear had come back entirely clear — had it been a small sample, or other difficulty? He looked at the report and said that these days if there were any queries they ask for a new smear.

"Mikki continued having pain and towards the end of October asked her GP to examine her. He found the growth — mainly on the side of the cervix rather in the middle where the smear is usually taken from. I knew from his gasp that it was serious and asked him to be honest — he said he thought it was a growth, and when I asked for his opinion he told me he thought it was a large cancer.

"She saw a gynaecologist who referred her for a colposcopy examination, but not until 5th November. When she wrote to me she had just seen the oncologist.

"The gynaecologist was not at all helpful, and gave me no new information. My own GP had the biopsy analysed quickly, which showed an aggressively growing irregular cancer. I saw the oncologist on Monday of this week, who confirmed my, and my GP's, fears that the pain in my back could be the cancer spreading. I am on an emotional roller coaster that I know you will recognise. The oncologist (as opposed to the gynaecologist) is someone who explains things, but also does not give heaps of information which you could not possibly take in."

I spoke to Mikki on the phone after receiving her letter. She told me she was receiving a lot of support from her colleagues — she worked in the Social Services Department. She also mentioned that she had a professional relationship with many medical staff which made talking to them easier for her than it might be for other women.

When Mikki wrote again, at the end of January 1997, she had just completed a second batch of radiotherapy treatments. She wrote:

"I think that I have already relayed some experiences in my letter to you. I am happy that you use or disregard any or all of that. I have also put some observations below — forgive me if I'm repeating myself!

"The biggest thing for me, and on which I will now try and educate all the GPs in my area, is that the medical profession appear to rely too heavily on the reliability of smears. If that had not been the case mine could have been picked up at least a little earlier — my GP could have examined me sooner, and the scan should have been investigated rather than assuming it showed a fibroid because my smear was clear.

"My family and my husband have been very supportive and I have been touched and amazed by the response, not only of close colleagues, but also of people from other agencies and organisations that I have worked with. I attended my team's Christmas party and to begin with they were not sure what to say to me.

"Emotionally, I have been very up and down. At times I have felt (and may do in the future) that there isn't any point in fighting as it will get me in the end — at other times when it is going well I am elated. I have just finished my DMS/NVQ5, and will be starting back to work in February. I have leave owing so will do a three day week through February and March and have booked a holiday in April!"

Following this letter, I did not hear from Mikki again. I sent her regular up-dates on my progress with the book, as I did all to contributors. One sunny afternoon in May I received a telephone call from Mikki's husband, who simply said: "My wife died just last week."

I was stunned and speechless. All the people who have so frankly shared their experiences have become like old friends to me. I was not able to say anything very much that day. I later wrote saying how sorry I was, and asking permission to dedicate this book to Mikki. We have kept in touch since then, and Brian has very kindly made a donation towards the publishing costs of the book.

I had been agonising over whether to include 'Mikki's story' in this book, as she cannot approve the final copy the way everyone else has. But, with her husband's permission, and given her expressed approval above, we have decided one way to honour her wish to spread awareness of the importance of being aware of and investigating symptoms, is to include her account. I have also received a contribution from Carol, Mikki's close friend and work colleague. We hope that Mikki's story will help people to be able to find ways to live the life they want when the prognosis is bad — it means a great deal that the quality of the last months of life are as good as possible.

Brian's story

After Brian had approved the account above, he sent me these words to be included:

I'm 43 years old. Mikki was 42. We had been married for 13 years, but we knew each other from our college days. It is not easy to put into words how one feels at the loss of your partner who you thought would be with you well into your old age. Your life grinds to a halt, you are left alone with no one to share your thoughts with, or to talk to about the day's events.

Mikki was a very brave person, never complaining, always putting on a smile even when she was in great pain. Due to the nature of her work, and that of her colleagues, she knew the outcome was not going to be good.

When Mikki first told me the diagnosis in October 1996, after she had visited the doctor, I thought: "Hey, a bit of radiation, and it will be OK." Sadly, that was not to be. The pain she went through, aching back, swollen legs, loss of weight, vomiting, constant visits to the toilet, was hard for both of us. Many a night I would wake up to the sound of Mikki crying with pain. All I could do was to hold her close to me, comforting her, both wishing the pain to go away, still hoping the treatment would work and end this nightmare.

In April 1997 we went on holiday for a week with the doctor's consent, taking half a suitcase full of tablets to ease Mikki's pain. The holiday was a good break, Mikki was able to go horse-riding, her favourite pastime, and I played some golf.

Just two weeks later, Mikki was taken to hospital where she died on 10th May 1997.

May I thank Mary Lunnen for dedicating this book to Mikki. Also thank you to everybody involved in the book, both in contributing their stories, and helping with publication. On a personal note may I say:

"Mikki - there's no goodbyes, just good memories."

My friend Mikki - Carol's story

Mikki was my friend, my best friend. She was also my boss. Not an easy combination, but one which worked well for us. I think we were always honest with each other both at work and leisure. At work she was always the boss and I respected her knowledge, skills, and her ability to be both a strong manager and a compassionate human being.

At leisure she could be crazy and she played hard, often pushing herself. We used to go horse riding, and walking our dogs. We both enjoyed training our dogs in obedience and agility clubs.

When she first started to feel ill in May and June 1996 I believe she had concerns that it was not a simple issue. Her clear smear test in July initially allayed some fears. I know she was really worried because she talked to me about the pain she had in her back — unlike her to complain.

She continued to work, but her pain, and the drugs she was taking, made some days a real struggle. The uncertainty and worry about the cause of her pain continued into

October. The diagnosis was the hardest thing to hear from her, and I remember that she chose her own time to tell me.

I arrived for one of our regular Sunday walks in the local woods. She told me that at last she had been given a positive diagnosis — of cervical cancer. We cried together and held each other. We both worked closely with disabled and terminally ill people so I think we both had thoughts of what may be.

We continued to walk together with our dogs, and we trained the dogs twice a week. All the time she was receiving radiotherapy and had to take increasingly powerful painkillers. I now believe that she remained positive for her family and her friends when she knew by February 1997 that no further treatment was possible.

She returned to work in February 1997 and her determination kept her going for four weeks but the pain was beginning to increase and she had to resort to steroids. She knew that staff and friends found it difficult to know what to say. We were able to talk about this but we had no answers. Her determination to continue to do all the things she valued was magnificent. She needed, as always, to feel in control.

The holiday she had in April with Brian and her friends, Caroline and Alan, was something she really looked forward to. Her pain was bad and the week before she went away it was touch and go as she needed to be able to get medical support urgently. Having the morphine to inject if necessary gave her confidence and she went away and had a wonderful time. She had to rest though, and this was so unlike her. Her energy was legendary, as was her capacity to do several things at once.

She did not return to work, and the steroids were making her feel uncomfortable. She did, however, still walk with me and our dogs, and attend almost all of our dog training sessions. Her colleagues at work visited her and were all aware that she was very ill, although she was determined not to give in.

In the last week of her life everything continued as usual, we went to the woods on Sunday, but instead of us walking, I drove us there and back. She was getting very breathless but we still went dog training on Tuesday night. On Wednesday I saw her in Canterbury when she and Brian took their dog to the vet for his injections. We were side by side in a traffic jam and talked through the car windows. On Thursday afternoon she went to the doctor's and I believe she knew she was beginning to run out of time. She was very anaemic and tired. She phoned me when she got home and said she and Brian were going out for a meal so she wouldn't be going to the dog agility training that night.

Next morning her doctor called at the house. She was very unwell and needed the boost of a blood transfusion. When Brian left for work at lunchtime she was resting but seemed OK. When he returned home she was very ill and in pain. She was admitted to hospital and was virtually unconscious. Brian rang me to let me know that the next morning, Saturday, they were going to try a blood transfusion. Mikki's mum stayed at the hospital as she could not bear to leave her. On Saturday morning Brian rang me at 9 a.m. to tell me that if I wanted to say goodbye to Mikki I would need to come to the hospital now.

I arrived at about 10 a.m., having rung Mikki's friends, Alan and Caroline, in Leicestershire. Mikki was unconscious. I stayed till 1.15 p.m. Caroline and Alan had arrived and I said my goodbyes to my friend. I arrived home and rang her friends at work so that they too could say goodbye. Mikki died before her colleagues could arrive at the hospital.

She had been in control until the last 24 hours of her life. I believe that this is how she would have wished it. I know she would not have wanted to be helpless and not in control of her destiny.

She was a good and loyal friend and I miss her now, ten months on, as much as I missed her then. She has left a space in my life and my heart that it is impossible to fill. I hope to carry on with some of the work she started with the protection of vulnerable adults. This will help me to move on.

When we were together we talked a lot. When she wasn't at work she wanted me to tell her what was going on. She hated it if I didn't talk straight. She didn't want to hear only the good things. When I had problems she didn't always try to make it better, but she used to think about situations when we were apart and she would ring me up with advice or suggestions.

We had times when we talked about her illness. She often found it difficult to admit to the level of pain she was in. She seemed to need to protect those around her. Holding her hand one Sunday morning in February when she had had a severe episode of pain gave me an insight into her need to keep in control, and that the pain temporarily prevented this. She was angry at this and frightened. We had both worked with people who relied on doctors to help them control pain and we did have faith that this was possible. What Mikki hated was that the analgesics often made her sleepy, and nearly stopped her carrying on with her life.

People who know me know that silence is something I find hard to cope with. During the time I was privileged to be with Mikki, I found how valuable silence can be if you are with someone you trust and value. When we talked it was always about living — what we were planning with the dogs, the impending birth of my grandson. I believe now that she did this to help me. She knew what was to come but she didn't want pity and I believe she wanted to protect those around her. I know that she talked to an aunt and to support groups about the prognosis. I am glad she did this. She found it easier to be honest about her fears with people she didn't see every day.

Mikki lived life to the full over the last six months of her life. This was how she wanted it. Mostly she remained in control. After her death Brain and I found post-it notes to us in unexpected places. They contained messages to us. One of mine was how to plant and cultivate a Magnolia tree. We both loved the plant and now I have one in my garden which will always remind me of her. She had less than 24 hours in hospital and by then she was already unconscious. She did not suffer the indignity of helplessness, which I know she would have hated.

Mikki was a very brave lady who won the respect of all of the people who worked with her and the love of many more.

Last thoughts - lessons to be learned

Reading through these accounts of battles against cancer, all sorts of issues emerge. It is extraordinary and shocking that 3 out of 15 women first learned that they had cancer by receiving an appointment card for radiotherapy treatment. It is to be hoped that this will not continue to happen in the future.

A life-threatening illness may lead to a total change in our aims, or a realisation of what is really important to us which may have been obscured by the pressures of normal day-to-day living, which for many women is a continuous juggling act with no time for reflection. Facing the possibility of death strips away all the clutter and leaves no time for niceties. Many of us have become more impatient with those things that waste time and are not essential, and have come to appreciate fully those things that are really important to us.

Several themes emerge through the telling of these stories:

• that it is vital for women to take advantage of regular smear tests.

• the importance of the knowledge to be aware of the early symptoms of cervical cancer rather than relying solely on smear test results.

• the difficulty of obtaining full information from the doctors - their reluctance to use the word 'cancer' and make clear exactly what is involved in treatment.

• the inadequate and sometimes insensitive way in which the news is given (in spite of changes in approaches by some clinicians).

• the lack of information available about complementary therapies, which while not replacing 'standard' medicine, can provide real benefits.

• facing up to the possibility of death can lead us to make positive changes in the way we live our lives.

The use of smear tests for screening for cancer is vital. Although the recent scandals indicate that the accuracy and reliability of these need to be improved, the experiences described here show that the current system can be invaluable in making an early diagnosis and in saving lives. New developments such as computer analysis of smear tests appear to have potential for reducing the possibility of errors. According to recent figures, of over 4 million smears examined last year in the UK, 8.6% of the valid tests (i.e. around 30,000) were found to have abnormalities. (Source: *DoH Statistical bulletin* 1997/27). Deaths in the same time from cervical cancer were around 1400, and many lives must have been saved by early diagnosis from the screening service.

Communications between clinicians and patients are so important. Even though this is recognised to a greater extent today, the pressures of time and resources mean that doctors, both GPs and hospital consultants, have little time to spend with their patients. In my opinion this could be a false economy, as giving doctors more time to treat their patients as people, and really listen to them, could pay off in reduced costs of treatment. Many people feel real anger at the way they have been treated during their illness. This may be for various reasons: slow or mis-diagnosis, faults in smear tests, insensitive treatment.

The old attitudes to cancer remain — as something that has to be spoken of in a whisper. Cervical cancer in particular was seen as something shameful, that must somehow be the woman's fault. As with many cancers, it is not known what causes cervical cancer. Risk factors quoted include the human papilloma virus (HPV), smoking, long-term use of the contraceptive pill, early sexual activity, many sexual partners. These are not proven causes, and may be associated with each other rather than with the risk of cervical cancer itself. (For a very clear explanation of the issues see Dr Anne Szarewski: *The Cervical Smear Test*). The fact that these are stated in various publications contributes to the stigma that still attaches to a diagnosis of cervical cancer.

However, it is possible for women with none of these factors to contract the disease, and equally of course, many others do not contract it in spite of one or several being present. Dr William M Rich (Clinical Professor of Obstetrics and Gynaecology, University of California, San Francisco) mentions, in an article published on the Internet, that:

'All sexually active women are at risk for the development of cervical cancer. The risk seems to be increased with smoking and promiscuity of the woman or her male partner. This is the standard text book explanation for an increased risk. But, in my experience, it is not a likely explanation for the patients that I have treated. It is not increased by the use of birth control pills, family history or the development of genital warts. Almost all cases occur in women who have not had regular screening with Pap (cervical smear) tests. This is one cancer that can be prevented, in most cases, by screening for the premalignant changes.'

Peggy Foster, in *Women and the Health Care Industry; an unhealthy relationship?*, discusses cervical cancer screening, and quotes a researcher, Peter Skrabnek, who says that the links that researchers, epidemiologists and doctors have constantly made between female promiscuity and cervical cancer are not only sexist and degrading but virtually meaningless: "It seems that promiscuity, if it means anything, is having more sex than the investigator!" Peggy Foster goes on to say that: "experts in the field continue to refer to the 'risky' sexual behaviour of young girls, and continue, on the most part, to ignore the role of men in causing cervical cancer."

Sandra Coney in *The Menopause Industry*, provides a down-to-earth discussion of these issues, and mentions that even if cervical cancer is related to a sexually transmitted virus, this could have taken place years earlier: "It does not mean that either (partner) has been promiscuous or unfaithful, just normal human beings!". She also points out that adenocarcinomas (about 10% of cases) are not related to sexual intercourse at all. It is often more difficult for adenocarcinomas to be detected by a routine smear test. Dr Anne Szarewski provides a clear explanation of the different types of cervical cancer.

So, there really is no need for women diagnosed with cervical cancer to torture themselves with thoughts that they are in some way being 'punished' for things that may have happened in the past. It is more important to develop a positive and healthy attitude to the lives we are living now, and so do our best to contribute to our future good health.

In practical terms, the screening programme and greater awareness of symptoms mean that cervical cancer is no longer so much to be feared, and is becoming more and more survivable. Again and again the stories here emphasise the importance of awareness, not only amongst women but also amongst medical staff, of the value, but also the limitations, of smear testing.

The contributors to this book have ideas and suggestions to help women once they have been diagnosed. These cover things such as dealing with the worries of family and friends, coping with side-effects, re-evaluating your priorities in life. (see Appendix 1 which provides a summary of some of these points from the stories).

Along with most of the writers here, I felt totally alone when I was told I had cervical cancer. I myself feel that I may have coped better if I had had the chance to talk to other patients. As mentioned by Helen, all patients undergoing treatment for cancer can be a great support for each other. If I had realised this at the time I may have contacted a cancer group, though there was not an active group near to my home.

Some contributors have reported that the general groups did not seem very relevant to their particular cases. However, many groups are obviously a marvellous support to their members, witness the description given by Bernadette of the meetings she attends. There are also some specialised groups such as Gynae-C, and others listed in Appendix 2. The specialist cancer nurses who answer the CancerBACUP lines are able to provide information on all aspects of cancer. They are also there to listen to all the worries or troubles of patients and their families. This service was important to me, and I hope that this book will also help relieve the feelings of many of us when diagnosed that we are the only person in the world to have this disease.

One of the reasons why I, and so many of the contributors to this book have found complementary therapies so beneficial is that practitioners in these areas are taught that a vital part of the treatment is listening to the person they are treating. This means treating them as a whole person, not as an example of a disease. The acupuncturist who helped me a great deal is a GP. We talked in some depth about a wide range of issues during my sessions with him. One of the things he told me was that he disliked working full-time in the NHS because of the pressure to rush patients in and out of his surgery in ten minutes.

As well as treating symptoms and pain relating to cancer and its medical treatments, complementary medicine can help us to stay well by teaching healthy ways of living, and healthy attitudes. The techniques of relaxation, affirmations and visualisation that are so useful for cancer patients, are valuable ways of coping with everyday life. Appendix 2 includes some contact addresses for various organisations which register recognised practitioners, and Appendix 3 has some books listed covering complementary medicine. I have found Bernie Siegal's books (*Love, Medicine and Miracles* and *Peace, Love and Healing*) both convincing and inspiring, written as they are by someone educated to take a scientific approach.

The experience of being told that you have cancer is something no one could possibly wish for, but once it has happened, if you can treat it as an experience that can be learnt from, it is possible eventually to leave it behind in the past. This is something that can take many years to really work through. I personally hate the expressions 'come to terms with', and 'learn to live with', as I have most often heard them used in a rather condescending tone by doctors. It always seemed to me that doing this implied putting up with second best all the time. However there is some truth in those sayings, in that the only way to continue life and not let the horrors of the past haunt you is not to forget, but to use these experiences in an active way.

This is extremely difficult and all of us have our own ways of coping. Some of the people whose stories you have read here have made major changes in their lives, others have adapted more gradually to what has happened to them. Some have continued with their previous careers with more enthusiasm and joy for living. Some have changed jobs, husbands, style of living totally. Some have become involved in helping others such as Helen with the Gynae-C helpline, and myself in compiling this book.

Positive thinking is a way of looking at life which can help everyone, not only cancer patients, enjoy every minute of their daily life as much as possible. This may sound unrealistically cheery, and I am myself somewhat inclined to what the Victorians would have called 'melancholy'. However having 'practised' (with a struggle at times) positive thinking for some time now, I do find it becomes easier to recover from the black days that we all have when everything goes wrong and life doesn't seem worth living. One of the books I have found very useful is *You can heal your Life*, by Louise L. Hay, though I have found that the 'right' time for me to read it has only been very recently, nearly four years after my diagnosis. Other favourite books of mine are listed in Appendix 3, all of which may contain nuggets that will ring true for you at a particular moment, even if all the ideas are not useful or relevant.

I feel I am at last beginning to develop a new approach to life in which every moment is precious. I try to take time to appreciate every day and notice the amazing things around us even in humdrum settings. If we do not believe in life after death, the old saying: 'life is not a rehearsal' — inspires us to make the best of every moment if we possibly can. For those of us who do have the view that there is something else to follow, experiences, positive or negative, are sent so that we may learn from them and develop as individuals. In either case I believe that the power of love is just the most important influence in the world, if you can concentrate on that everything else slips into place.

Looking back at the stories in this book, love and laughter are the two things have got all of us through the bad times. The support of families and friends - just being there when we needed them, the children (our own or other people's) who we hope to see grow up, the sheer determination not to be beaten by the 'silent but deadly disease' (to quote Pauline) — are all things that have kept us going.

It is a big step to face up to the prospect of your own death, but it is something everyone has to do at some time, so maybe we are lucky. Once we have been through an experience such as ours, it makes everyday life more precious, and helps us to be content in the little moments that added together make a lifetime. If we are forever yearning for the 'better' things we hope will come tomorrow, we can miss the joys around us today.

Each moment has the possibility of a new discovery. Yet, when it passes, that moment never returns. Only as I am aware of the present will I have the opportunity to be fully alive. Just a normal day — what a gift! (Anne Wilson Schaef)

The Future

The writing of this book, which has taken nearly two years, has introduced me to many wonderful people, not only the contributors themselves, but many others who have helped and inspired me in all sorts of ways.

I plan to continue and develop the work on awareness begun here. Possible projects include producing packs for doctors and patients that could be widely distributed, giving not only contacts and practical advice, but also some of the personal stories as well. Other avenues include investigating further the various complementary therapies available; writing articles and attending, and speaking at, conferences, meetings etc. I have also discussed with the Centre for Complementary Health Studies at the University of Exeter the possibility of developing my work into a research proposal, which I hope will come to fruition at some time in the future. I also hope to continue to participate in the Research Forum of the Hypatia Trust* on 'Women and Cancer' topics.

I would welcome any correspondence from people interested in this work, please address to: Mary Lunnen, Manapouri, Treleigh Farm, Rumford, Wadebridge, Cornwall, PL27 7RT, Tel: 01841 540552, Email: mlunne@globalnet.co.uk

* The Hypatia Trust was established in 1996 to preserve and protect the women's history collections housed at the Jamieson Library at Newmill, Penzance and at Exeter University. The aim of the Trust is 'to further understanding of Woman and her achievements'. Its work is carried out through a series of teaching and learning forums and their publication, bound together in the Hypatia Institute. Contact: Melissa Hardie, The Hypatia Trust, The Old Post

Office, Newmill, Penzance, Cornwall, TR20 8XN. Tel: 01736 360549, FAX/Tel: 01736 333307, FAX: 01736 330704. E-mail: OldPostOfficeNewmill@compuserve.com. Websites: http//www.hypatia-trust.org.uk and http//www.ex.ac.uk//hypatia/

Glossary of technical terms

adnexa — adjoining parts, i.e. fallopian tubes and ovaries which adjoin the uterus.

adenocarcinoma — a malignant new growth of glandular epithelial tissue in its original position.

Alexander technique — a way of physical and mental tensions and improving posture.

aromotherapy — the use of essential oils from aromatic plants to assist and maintain health.

biopsy — removal of a small amount of tissue for microscopic examination.

carcinoma in situ — confirmed cancer in place.

catheter — narrow tube inserted into the bladder to drain it, attached to bag to collect urine.

cervical erosion — extension of cells to outer part from inner part of cervix.

colposcopy — examination of the cervix using a colposcope (similar to a small microscope). The cervix is painted with a solution to show up the areas of abnormal cells. A loop diathermy may be undertaken at the same time to remove abnormal cells.

colostomy — surgical operation to bring colon through abdominal wall to create an opening or 'stoma'.

cone biopsy — a cone-shaped section of the cervix is removed under general anaesthetic when the abnormal cells cannot be seen clearly with the colposcope.

CT (or CAT) scan — Computerised (Anatomical) Tomography. A development of diagnostic radiology, records 'slices' of the soft tissues of the body.

D & C— 'dilation and curettage': cervix is stretched open ('dilated') and lining of uterus removed ('curettage').

diagnostic cystoscopy — examination of the urinary bladder with instrument via urethra.

diathermy — heat, generated by electrical apparatus, to coagulate blood and destroy tissues.

episiotomy — incision to enlarge vaginal opening.

EUA — Examination Under Anaesthetic.

fibroid — benign lump of fibrous tissue growing in uterus.

hysteroscopy — examination, with light source, of interior of uterus.

histology — study of tissue structures with light and microscope.

HRT — Hormone Replacement Therapy: in tablet form, or as patches, to replace hormones no longer produced when ovaries are removed or damaged by radiotherapy.

hysterectomy — **Wertheim's hysterectomy** where the uterus, ovaries, lymph nodes, and the upper part of the vagina are removed. **2)- radical** -- a non-specific term, usually used to mean ovaries and uterus are removed.

kinesiology — A system of assessing and restoring the body's energy flows. Includes 'zero balancing' to correct muscle alignments.

laparoscopy — Examination of organs of pelvis using a surgical instrument inserted through a small abdominal incision.

loop diathermy — uses heat to remove abnormal cells, under local anaesthetic.

lymph nodes — filter the lymph (fluid) which bathes the tissues. Also produce lymphocytes (white blood cells).

lymphodema — accumulation of lymph in the tissues.

MRI scan — Magnetic Resonance Imaging: 'maps' variation in tissues.

ovarian cyst — fluid-filled sac which develops in the ovary.

pelvic exenteration — surgical removal of lower abdominal contents.

polycystic ovaries — multiple cysts in the ovaries — hormonal disorder.

Reiki healing — healing based on eastern principles of healing technique, personal development, spiritual discipline, and mystic order.

reflexology — a precise form of therapeutic foot massage which promotes good health by relieving stress and tension, and restoring vital energy flow to the body.

speculum — metal instrument to hold cavity open for interior examination.

squamous — flat surface cells.

tai chi — Chinese system of gentle exercise movements.

urostomy — surgical operation to bring urethra through abdominal wall to create an opening.

uterus — womb.

venflon — the means of passing anaesthetic or drugs into the blood stream of the patient, normally attached to the back of the hand.

visualisation — a method of bringing happy relaxed pictures to mind, to block pain, discomfort and anxiety.

zero balancing — correction of muscle imbalance diagnosed by kinesiology by various techniques including acupressure, massage, exercises.

Appendix 1 — Practical Advice

As you will have seen throughout the book, the contributors' stories contain advice for other people to use when going through similar experiences. The main points are summarised below.

For all women:
* it is vital for women to take advantage of regular smear tests.
* the importance of the knowledge to be aware of the early symptoms of cervical cancer rather than relying solely on smear test results. These are:
* bleeding between periods (especially after intercourse)
* discharge
* discomfort.

Following diagnosis:
* get as much information as you can, take notes, arrange to contact someone to ask questions later, etc.
* take someone with you to consultations to give you moral support and ask questions for you.
* do as much as possible to feel you are in control of what is happening to you.
* get reading matter (e.g. from CancerBACUP and libraries).
* talk to people,
* investigate complementary therapies which may help you.
* organise help with domestic work for when treatment begins.

Following surgery:
- take the advice to rest as much as possible.
- build up activities very gradually, spend a short time on anything and stop if it becomes too painful or tiring.
- give yourself plenty of treats and things to look forward to - good books, outings, chats on the phone.

During and following radiotherapy:
- organise a rota of friends and family to drive to treatment sessions with you.
- practice visualisation techniques.

Be aware that long-term effects of treatment can include:
- pain
- exhaustion
- fluid retention, lymphdoema
- numbness, caused by cutting of nerves during surgery, feeling usually returns gradually
- disturbed sleep patterns.

General advice:
- pamper yourself.
- give yourself as much rest as is needed.
- when in pain, pace yourself, really rest between each effort if this is necessary.
- continue with healthy diet, and complementary therapies that help you.
- talk to others who have similar experiences if possible. Sharing and humour always help!

Advice for and from family members:
- make life as normal as possible, one of the worst things is being treated as a patient.
- be prepared to listen to worries, and talk about feelings - something you may not normally do.

- expect mood swings and tears.
- help in finding practical advice, and allow the person to be in control as much (or little) as they want.
- be aware that the effects of having cancer last a long time after apparent recovery.
- seek help for yourself - someone to talk about your worries and fears. CancerBACUP can help with this.

Appendix 2 - contact addresses

General Cancer Organisations

CancerBACUP, 3 Bath Place, Rivington Street, London, EC2A 3JR. Freeline: 080018 11 99, Cancer Information Service: 0171 613 2121

Cancer Counselling Service: 0171 696 9000 (London) or 0141 553 1553 (Glasgow)

The free number above will be answered by a nurse with whom you can discuss anything you wish in confidence, and request further information and booklets. CancerBACUP also have an excellent Internet site at: http://www.cancerbacup.org.uk. This has an extensive database of organisations and support groups across the UK. Also details of publications and other resources. If you cannot access the Internet, the telephone number above will give contact details and information.

CancerLink, 11-21 Northdown Street, London, N1 9BN, 0171 833 2818

Cancer Care Society, 21 Zetland Road, Redland, Bristol, BS6 7AH, 0117 942 7419 or 0117 923 2302

Cancer Relief Macmillan Fund, Anchor House, 15-19 Britten Street, London, SW3 3TZ, 0171 351 7811

Marie Curie Cancer Care, 28 Belgrave Square, London, SW1X 8QG, 0171 201 2330 or 0171 235 3325

Northumberland Cancer Support Group*, Linda Brinkhurst (Secretary/Chairman), 47 Apperley Road, Stocksfield, Northumberland, 01661 842919

North Ayrshire Cancer Care*, Muirside Lodge, Stevenson Road, Kilwinning, Ayrshire, Scotland, 01294 552223/556550, Fax: 01294 551440

*there are local groups all around the country, your GP, hospital, or Health Information service will be able to give you contact details.

Cervical cancer or other gynae cancers

Gynae-C, 1 Bolingbroke Road, Swindon, Wiltshire, SN2 2LB, 01793 480298

Abnormal Smear Care Group, Linda Brown, c/o Community House, 173 Derby Road, Long Eaton, Nottingham, NG10 4LL, 0115 946 8988 (address will be changing soon, but phone no. will remain the same.)

Durham Women's Cancer Group, Jo McLaughlin, 25 Browning Hill, Cixhoe, Durham, DH6 4HB, 0191 377 0541. Mainly breast cancer, but open to all women.

Dropin Centre, Carol Hancock , Ward 59, Clarendon Wing, Leeds General Infirmary, Leeds, West Yorkshire, 01132 922359. Open to any woman with gynaecological cancer regardless of where the cancer is diagnosed and/or treated.

Other useful addresses

General

British Complementary Medicine Association (BCMA), 39 Prestbury Road, Cheltenham, Glos., GL52 2PT, 01242 226770

British Holistic Medicine Association (BHMA), Rowlands Thomas House, Royal Shrewsbury Hospital South, Shrewsbury, Shropshire, SY3 8XF, 01743 261155.

Council for Complementary and Alternative Medicine (CCAM), 179 Gloucester Place, London, NW1 6DX, 0171 724 9103

Warwickshire Complementary Cancer Care, Mrs Gerry Bishop, Romilie, Eathorpe, Leamington Spa, Warwickshire, CV33 9DE, 01926 633353, Resource Centre open one Saturday per month.

Specific therapies

British Acupuncture Association and Register, 34 Alderly Street, Victoria, London, SW1V 4EU, 0171 834 1012.

British Medical Acupuncture Association (BMAS), 27a Devonshire Street, London, W1N 1RJ, 0171 935 2163.

British Herbal Medicine Association (BHMA), Field House, Lye Hole Lane, Redhill, Avon, BS18 7TB

British Homeopathic Association (BHA), 27a Devonshire Street, London, W1N 1RJ, 0171 935 2163.

British Wheel of Yoga, Central Office, 1 Hamilton Place, Boston Road, Sleaford, Lincs., NG34 7ES' 01529 306851

International Society of Professional Aromatherapists, 82 Ashby Road, Hinckley, Leics., LE10 1SE, 01455 637987.

National Federation of Spiritual Healers, Old Manor Farm Studio, Church Street, Sunbury on Thames, Middx., TW16 6RG, 01932 783164.

Healer referral service: 01891 616080

The Shiatsu Society, 5 Foxcote, Wokingham, Berks., RG11 3PG, 01734 730836

The Reiki Association, Contact: Kate Jones, Administrative Director, Cornbrook Bridge House, Cornbrook, Clee Hill, Ludlow, Shropshire, SY8 3QQ, Tel & Fax: 01584 891197

Appendix 3 - further reading and references

I have only included here books that I have read myself and found useful, most give further reading lists. There are many general publications on cancer, but I have found that the booklets supplied by CancerBACUP (and by other organisations such as Macmillan and CancerLink) are best as they are able to keep up-to-date with the latest research. They also include reading lists of further publications on each subject.

CancerBACUP

Free information booklets for patients include:

Understanding cervical smears

Understanding cancer of the cervix

Complementary therapies and cancer

Sexuality and cancer

What do I tell the children?

What now? Adjusting to life after cancer

Who can ever understand?-- talking about your cancer

Lost for words. How to talk to someone with cancer

Write for a full list to: CancerBACUP, 3 Bath Place, Rivington Street, London, EC2A 3JR, 0171 696 9003. CancerBACUP have an excellent web site on the Internet that includes the full text of all their booklets and many other resources such as contact details for organisations and groups around the UK: http://www.cancerbacup.org.uk.

Smear tests

Dr Anne Szareweski, *(A woman's guide to)The Cervical Smear Test*, Optima, 1994, ISBN 0-356-210332 £6.99. Comprehensive guide to the smear test, and cervical cancer, explaining medical terms.

Changing your life - inspiring books

Sandra Ban Breathnach, Simple Abundance — *A Daybook of Comfort and Joy*, Bantam Books, 1997 ISBN 0-553-50662-5. Appreciating the simple joys of life.

Julia Cameron, *The Artist's Way-- A course in discovering and recovering your creative self.*, Pan Books, 1995 ISBN 0330-34358-0. Ideas to nurture your creativity.

Anne Dickson, *A woman in your own right*, Quartet, 1982 ISBN 0-7043-3420-8, A classic assertiveness book.

Lynda Field, *Self-Esteem for Women*, Element, 1997 ISBN 1-85230-936-9.Includes exercises to help change the way you see yourself.

Betty Friedan, *The Fountain of Age*, Vintage, 1994 ISBN 0-09-916481-7. Argues for a different attitude to ageing, as a 'grand adventure'.

Wendy Grant, *Are you in control?*, Element, 1996 ISBN 1-85230-778-1. Overcoming fears, stress-management.

Louise L Hay, *You can heal your life*, Eden Grove Editions, 1996 IBSN 1-870845-21-8

Positive thinking, affirmations.

The Hen Co-op, *Disgracefully Yours*, Judy Piatkus, 1995 ISBN 0-7499-1472-6, Celebrating life!

Marlene E Hunter, *Making Peace with Chronic Pain -- A Whole-Life Strategy*, Brunner/Mazel, 1996 ISBN 0-87630-821-3, Techniques for dealing with pain

Nancy Kline, *Women and Power*, BBC Books, 1993 ISBN 0-563-36449-1, Creating a 'thinking environment' and support structures at work.

Elisabeth Kübler-Ross, *The Wheel of Life*, Bantam Press, 1997 ISBN 0593-043022, Extraordinary memoirs of the author of 'Death & Dying'.

Dr Christiane Northrup, *Women's Bodies, Women's Wisdom*, Piatkus, 1995 ISBN 0-7499-1484-X (pbk) Holistic approach to self-healing.

Stephan Rechtschaffen, *Time Shifting*, Rider, 1996 ISBN 0-7126-7282-6, Changing our perceptions of time, to make more of it for ourselves.

Anne Wilson Schaef, *Meditations for women who do too much*, HarperSanFranscisco, 1990 ISBN 0-06-254866-2, Meditations to help women break the cycle of doing too much.

Betty Shine, *Mind to Mind*, Corgi, 1994 ISBN 0-552-13378-7, Memoirs of a healer.

Betty Shine, *Betty Shine's Mind Workbook*, Corgi, 1994 ISBN 0-552-14214-X, Exercises and visualisations.

Bernie Siegel, *Love, Medicine and Miracles*, Arrow Books, 1989 ISBN 0-09-963270-5. Classic book on healing and the mind/body relationship, for patients and physicians.

Bernie Siegal, *Peace, Love and Healing*, Arrow Books, 1991 ISBN 0-09-974670-0. Follow-up to his first book, discusses scientific evidence for self-healing. Many inspiring stories.

Linda Valins, *Intimate Matters-- restoring harmony and balance to the feminine experience.*, Gaia Books, 1993 ISBN 1-85675-070-1. Creating a positive relationship between you and your body.

Discussion of healthcare issues

Sandra Coney, *The Menopause Industry*, The Women's Press, 1995 ISBN 0-7043-4398-3, Discussion of a range of women's health issues.

Anne Dickson & Nikki Henriques, *Hysterectomy -- the woman's view*, Quartet, 1994 ISBN 0-7043-0214-4. Excellent practical advice from professionals, and quotes from women with experience of hysterectomy.

Peggy Foster, *Women and the health care industry -- an unhealthy relationship?*, Open University Press, 1995 ISBN 0-333-09472-4 (pbk) A critical look at women's healthcare.

Books on experiences

Sandra Butler and Barbara Rosenblum, *Cancer in two voices*, The Women's Press, 1991 ISBN 0-7043-4393-2. Story of a woman's life and death with breast cancer.

Anne Dennison, *Uncertain Journey -- a woman's experience of living with cancer*, The Patten Press, 1996 ISBN 1-872229-23-9. Powerful account of Anne's experiences of terminal ovarian cancer.

Frances Ive, *Please don't die yet -- I'm not ready*, Five Press, 1997 ISBN 0-9531134-0-X. A personal account of losing both parents.

Audre Lorde, *The Audre Lorde Compendium*, Pandora, 1996 ISBN 0-04-440955-9. Extracts from the writings of the American feminist writer, including 'The Cancer Journals', her account of living with breast cancer.

Penny Snow, *A Referred Pain -- reflections on family life and cancer*, The Patten Press, 1997 ISBN 1-872229 -14-X. Reflections following the death of both Penny Snow's parents from cancer.

Liz Tilberis, *No Time to Die*, Weidenfield & Nicolson, 1998 ISBN 0 297 84236 6. Autobiography of the editor of Vogue and Harpers Bazaar, includes her fight with ovarian cancer, and discussion of latest research, though much of the book consists of inside tales of the fashion industry.